Physical Activity and the Older Adult
Psychological Perspectives

ANDREW C. OSTROW

West Virginia University

GV
482.6
.O84
1984

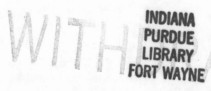

PRINCETON BOOK COMPANY, PUBLISHERS

PRINCETON, NEW JERSEY

jm
3-24-86

PHYSICAL ACTIVITY AND THE OLDER ADULT

Copyright © 1984 by
Princeton Book Company, Publishers
All rights reserved
Design by Bruce Campbell
Typesetting by Delmas

Library of Congress Catalog Card Number 83-063191
ISBN 916622-28-2
Printed in the United States of America

To Bella and Herman
&
Rebecca and Charles

who first taught me about the joys
and sorrows of growing old

Contents

Preface

This book is about the importance of remaining physically active as we grow older and the significance of physical activity in the lives of those who are old. When I was a boy growing up in Brooklyn, sports, games, and other forms of physical activity were an important part of my life. Playing punchball and stickball, jogging on the beach, or playing tennis over metal nets during the middle of winter were all important activities in my development. The vigor of activity, the sense of accomplishment, the thrill of victory, and the agonies of defeat left me with lasting memories. I was saddened to learn as I grew older that growing up often meant growing out of activity, and that new roles left little time for remaining physically active. Inevitably, I deduced that aging was synonymous with decline and that personal and social expectations made it "natural" for older people to refrain from participating in physical activity. Little did I realize that I was wrong.

This book explores the myths and realities of physical activity for the older adult. It is an appropriate textbook for upper-division and first-year graduate students who are taking courses related to gerontology, primarily in fields such as psychology, physical education, and life-span human development. Students in social work, nursing, and other allied health professions may find this textbook to be an important supplement to their training in gerontology. This textbook is also invaluable to those who are preparing to become leaders of older-adult physical activity programs.

The emphasis in this book is on evaluating the scientific evidence concerning the impact of physical activity on the physical and mental health of the older adult. Although the book primarily addresses the psychological concomitants of physical activity, gerontology, by definition, is an interdisciplinary endeavor. Thus, I have tried to weave knowledge from motor control and learning, exercise physiology, personality theory, sociology, and life-span development in order to better understand the role of physical activity in the lives of older adults.

Chapter 1 addresses the question of who is old and discusses the plight of the elderly in America. The potential of physical activity for ameliorating the conditions of being old is discussed. The chapter concludes by highlighting gerontology as a viable discipline worthy of academic pursuit.

Chapter 2 examines the research process, with special attention directed toward methodological concerns in studying aging processes and the older adult. Sampling considerations, measurement issues, and research design are important components of this chapter. These methodological concerns are illustrated by examining the research literature on the impact of physical activity on human life expectancy.

Chapter 3 focuses on age-related changes in physical fitness, psychomotor speed, and related personality variables. The overriding message in this chapter is that these changes may not only be inherent manifestations of biological aging, but may also be due to the increasingly sedentary life-styles we choose to follow as we grow older.

Chapter 4 explores this contention by examining what is known about the effects of exercise and other forms of physical activity on the physical and mental health of the older adult. This chapter presents evidence that the benefits of exercise and motor practice are not circumscribed by age and that older adults are trainable, even those who have been inactive for many years.

Unfortunately, in spite of the evidence documenting the benefits of physical activity, there appears to be a universal disengagement from physical activity as people grow older. Chapter 5 examines several social and psychological factors that may be partially responsible for our increasingly sedentary life-styles with advancing age.

Chapter 6 synthesizes information from previous chapters to present guidelines on the formulation of future programs of physical activity for the older adult. This chapter also discusses the training of physical activity leaders.

It was with a sense of urgency that I wrote this book. I am concerned that our current generation of older adults will be remembered as a forgotten and neglected generation who lived out their remaining years in poverty, desolation, and despair. As a physical educator, I feel that my profession and allied professions have much to offer that will help reduce the economic burden of medical care borne by the elderly and that will add vitality to their remaining years. Motor development is a lifelong process. The "graying of America" has forced many of us to reevaluate priorities that formerly have centered on a youth-oriented culture. Increasingly, there is the realization that physical activity must be promoted, pursued, and cherished throughout the life cycle.

Inevitably, the quality of a textbook extends far beyond the wisdom of its author. I am indebted to the principal reviewers of the manuscript, G. Lawrence Rarick, Professor Emeritus, University of California, Berkeley, Waneen Spirduso, Professor, University of Texas, Austin, and Matthew Kleinman, Associate Professor, Brooklyn College of CUNY for their extremely helpful suggestions and comments. I am also grateful to a number of my colleagues, William L. Alsop, J. William Douglas, Lucille Nahemow, Mary Kay White, and Robert L. Wiegand for their input on various portions of the manuscript. A special thanks to Carol Ann Straight, my typist, to Mark Fleming, my research assistant, and to Patricia Freedman, the copyeditor. I would be remiss if I did not also acknowledge the encouragement and assistance I received from Charles H. Woodford, President, Princeton Book Company, Publishers. Finally, I am deeply grateful to my family, Lynne, Jennifer, Olivia, Barney, Ruth, and Phil, whose love and devotion made the writing of this book all the more enjoyable.

Andrew C. Ostrow

1

Growing Old in America

Act I, Scene II of *The Nutcracker* opens as Dr. and Frau Silberhaus and their children welcome neighboring families to their home to share the splendor of Christmas Eve. Young children, parents, servants, and animated figures dance and frolic to the music of Tchaikovsky. Their movements are graceful, fluent, and vibrant. Suddenly, the children's grandparents emerge, excited by the festivities of the moment. Yet, they dance with trepidation, each step rigid, awkward, and painfully slow. Grandfather's sudden energetic dance movements seem to embarrass his wife and surprise the audience. This older couple leaves the stage, dizzy and gasping for air, as if apologetic for their sudden indulgence.

This scene symbolizes the theme of this book: understanding the role of physical activity* in the lives of older adults. Watching this older couple dance subtly reminds us of a number of important questions surrounding the myths and realities of remaining physically active as we grow older. Are slowness and rigidity of movement and increased cautiousness inevitable manifestations of the aging process? Why do many adults feel guilty and embarrassed about displaying feats of physical prowess when they are old? Why does society often characterize the elderly as listless and decrepit rather than as active and alive? What is known about the impact of physical activity on the mental health of older adults? These and other questions are the focus of this book.

WHO'S OLD?

The average life expectancy of Americans has jumped from 48 to 73 years since the turn of this century, primarily as a result of the eradication of many fatal childhood diseases, improved sanitation, and the promotion of other healthful practices. At the turn of the century, only 3.1 million Americans, or 4 percent of the population, were 65 years or older. Today, more than 25 million Americans (or 11 percent) are 65 years or older (U.S. Bureau of the Census, 1981). In 50 years, it is projected that 55 million

*The term *physical activity* can refer to an array of movement activities evident in the life experiences of older adults. For the purposes of this book, Kenyon's (1968) definition of physical activity as structured, nonutilitarian, gross human movement commonly manifested in sport, games, dance, and calisthenics will suffice.

1

Americans, or 18 percent of the population, will be over 65 years (Kalish, 1982).

The "graying of America" is a popular euphemism that reminds us that the median age of Americans is gradually increasing. Today, the median age of Americans is 30 years; it is estimated that the median age will have increased to 38 years in 2030. Individuals 65 years or older represent the fastest-growing age segment in the United States. There are currently 9.5 million Americans over 75 and 2.3 million Americans 85 years or older. By 2030, the 75-plus group will represent 40 percent of the elderly population ("American population," 1981).

Is there really a consensus, however, as to who is old in America? Historically, the age of 65 has been used to differentiate middle age from old age. This age has been used as a social convenience—65 had been mandated by the government as the age at which one retired (although recent laws have raised the age to 70), and many social services (such as Social Security) have been dictated by this age. However, even a cursory observation of older persons will reveal that people do not suddenly become old at the age of 65, and that there are large individual differences in the aging process.

Individual Differences

A consistent theme in the gerontological literature (e.g., Butler, 1975; Kalish, 1982) is that older people are more diverse than similar and that, with increasing age, there is greater variability in biological and behavioral functioning. Large *interindividual* differences exist among older persons on a number of personality and psychomotor parameters. Consequently, with advancing age, it becomes increasingly difficult to predict psychomotor performance and behavior using chronological age as the sole criterion. Nevertheless, chronological age has been used as an indicator of the physical, psychological, and social status of older persons (Butler, 1975). For example, Neugarten (1975) classified the "young-old" as individuals 55–75 years of age and the "old-old" as individuals over 75. The former group is generally healthier and its ratio of women to men is more equal. Shephard (1978) proposed a more elaborate classification scheme:

- Middle age—ages 40–65, the preretirement years
- Old age—ages 65–75, the immediate postretirement period when there is relatively minimal functional impairment
- Very old age—ages 75–85, some functional impairment but most individuals can still live somewhat independently
- Extreme old age—ages 85 and older, greater functional impairment and institutional care is usually needed

2

Chronological age classifications are, at best, convenient labels which help identify who is old. However, these labels may be somewhat simplistic in view of large cultural variations in the definition of who is old. In Japan, where age is revered, there is a movement toward raising the mandatory retirement age in the private sector from 55 to 60. In the Soviet Union, an acute labor shortage tends to discourage early retirement. However, in Kenya, where youth unemployment is rampant, youngsters are demanding that the compulsory retirement age be dropped to 50 or 45. While this may seem outrageous, a Nairobi law clerk was quoted as saying that it was better than the custom in Kenya 100 years ago when old, sick men were carried from their huts into the bush to be eaten alive by hyenas ("Now, the revolt," 1977).

Defined age categories are sometimes quite numerous across cultures. For example, the Comanche Indians distinguish 5 categories, the Kikuyu of Kenya have 6 categories for men and 8 for women, and the Andaman Islanders have 23 categories for men. These age categories are almost always associated with specific roles, statuses, and normative expectations (Falk, Falk, & Tomashevich, 1981).

The use of age categories also fails to consider that individuals do not age at the same rate—that is, there are large *intraindividual* differences in the aging process. Until now, I have used the term *aging* as if there were consensus as to how aging should be defined. For example, Birren and Renner (1977) suggested that "aging refers to the regular changes that occur in mature genetically representative organisms living under representative environmental conditions as they advance in chronological age" (p. 4). However, as Butler (1978) pointed out, it is important to remember that the study of aging is not just the study of diseases, disability, and decline; rather, it is the study of the normal processes of development.

Gerontologists recognize that being old can be translated into physical changes, behaviorial changes, and changes in social roles. Thus, efforts have been made toward describing the broad processes of aging in terms of *biological age,* or the functional capacities of our life-limiting organ systems; *psychological age,* or our functional and adaptive capacities toward environmental stimuli; and *social age,* or the roles and habits we exhibit with respect to other members of our community and society (Birren & Renner, 1977). Social, psychological, and biological changes that occur across the life cycle are often discontinuous rather than continuous and diverse rather than uniform.

There are many different rates of aging in the same individual. Thus, we often err in labeling individuals as old because of their physical appearance, forgetting that their psychological and social capacities for adaptation and change may be similar to (or more advanced) than people

3

half their age. Joe Hildebrand, professor emeritus of chemistry at the University of California, Berkeley, continues to publish and make major contributions to chemistry at the age of 100. He stated that he enjoyed skiing but his legs no longer obey him. "I am probably dying from my feet upward, which is better than starting at the top" (McDonald, 1981, p. 2).

Demographic Trends

As mentioned earlier, the median age of Americans is gradually increasing. People over 65 represent the fastest-growing segment of the U.S. population (see Table 1-1). When gerontologists study groups of aging individuals, they often use the term *cohort*. A cohort is a group of individuals sharing "similar" birthdates, and thus supposedly sharing a potentially unique set of social and cultural experiences that may differentially affect subsequent aging processes. For example, the large post–World War II "baby boom" produced a cohort that has had a remarkable impact on the vitality of our country. The 1960's and early 1970's witnessed a youth-oriented culture marked by liberalism and dissent. This cohort precipitated changes in our fashion industry, physical appearance, educational teaching practices, interpretations of

Table 1-1
Estimated Total U.S. Population 1970-1980-1990 by Age Groups
(in millions and percentages)

Year	0–19	20–34	Age group 35–49	50–64	65+
1970	76.8	45.6	34.8	30.7	20.9
	37%	22%	17%	14%	10%
1980	69.5	61.2	40.2	43.8	36.3
	29%	25%	17%	13%	16%
1990	64.5	62.2	51.5	35.8	51
	24%	23%	20%	14%	19%
1970–80 % change	−10	+34	+15	+7	+73
1980–90 % change	−7	−1.5	+28	+9	+40
1970–90 % change	−16	+36	+48	+16	+144

Note. Adapted from "Population Dynamics and Demography" by A.H. Underhill, *Journal of Physical Education, Recreation, and Dance*, 1981, *52*, 33-34. Reprinted by permission of the American Alliance for Health, Physical Education, Recreation, and Dance, 1900 Association Drive, Reston, VA 22091.

war heroes, sexual mores, and attitudes toward women and minority groups. This same cohort has also begun to question the future solvency of our Social Security system and the historic prejudices that have been exhibited toward the old.

There are several important demographic trends worthy of note when considering physical activity and the elderly. For example, until age 65 there is a gradual increase in the ratio of American women to men in 1980 as a function of chronological age; after 65, there are dramatic increases in the ratios of women to men (see Figure 1-1). These trends are remarkably similar to the data reported by Botwinick (1978) for 1970. Thus, it would appear that women (rather than men) may be the primary clientele of those conducting physical activity programs for older groups.

Interestingly, most men 65 and over are married; only one out of seven is widowed and only one out of seven lives alone. By contrast, more than 50 percent of women 65 and over are widowed, and more than a third of the women live alone; only one-third of women in this age group are married and living with their husbands (Murphy & Florio, 1978). These statistics may have important implications for organizing physical activity programs for the elderly.

The level of education of older adults continues to rise. For example, in 1952, only 18 percent of Americans aged 65 years or older had completed high school. Today, that figure is 38 percent, and by 1990 it is estimated that one-half of our older population will be high-school graduates (Watkins, 1981).

A common myth is that many older Americans are incapacitated and that most people over 65 are institutionalized. However, only 4 percent of those over 65 are institutionalized, with this figure approaching 17 percent among people over 85 (Botwinick, 1978). Most Americans under 85 are fully ambulatory (Clark, 1978) and quite capable of participating in programs of physical activity, if guidelines regulating the participation of these older adults in physical activity are carefully followed.

The distribution of the elderly across the United States shows more rapid gains in the elderly populations of our southern and western states (see Figure 1-2). Data indicate a movement of our retired population from the densely populated industrial states of the North and East to the warm climates and lower taxes of the South and West. Florida contains the highest percentage (14.6) of elderly residents over 65, and the greatest number of elderly (2.2 million) is found in California. Alaska claims the lowest percentage (2.3) of elderly residents (Fenstermacher, 1981). Thus, one could speculate that employment opportunities for individuals interested in developing physical activity programs for our elderly will be particularly prominent in the southern and western regions of the United States.

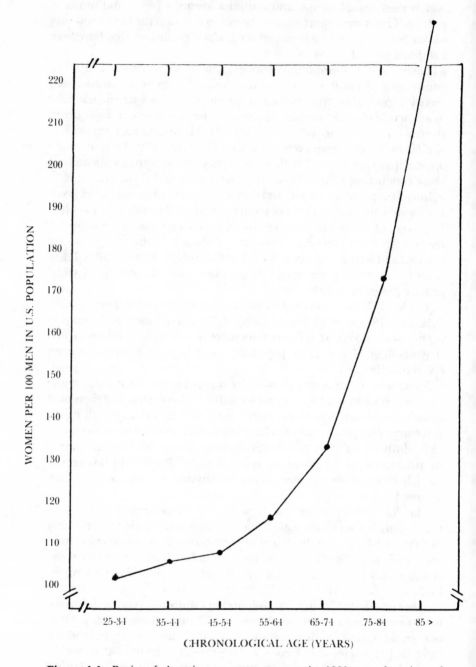

Figure 1-1. Ratio of American women to men in 1980 as a function of chronological age. (Data are from U.S. Bureau of the Census, 1981.)

6

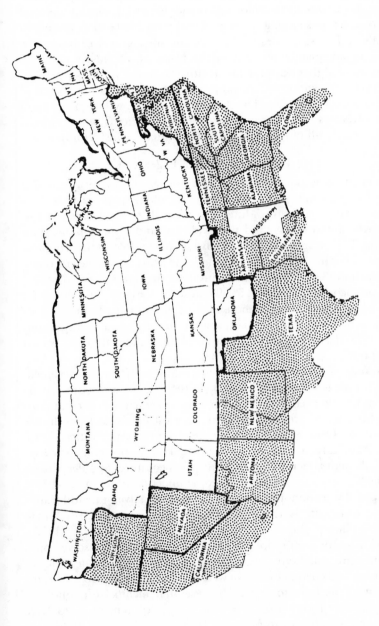

Figure 1-2. Distribution of elderly population in the United States. Shaded areas indicate states where elderly population grew at rate greater than U.S. average from 1960 to 1970. (From Fenstermacher, G.C. Elderly sunbelt migrants. *Journal of Physical Education, Recreation, and Dance,* 1981, 52, 57. Reprinted by permission of the American Alliance for Health, Physical Education, Recreation, and Dance, 1900 Association Drive, Reston, VA 22091.)

The data presented here provide evidence for a rapidly expanding elderly population in which women predominate and which is on the move to the warm regions of our country. The implications of these demographic trends are enormous. Demands for social, educational, and recreational services among the elderly will probably be more evident in the Sunbelt. Tax structures of the states in this region will have to be adjusted to adequately respond to the needs of an elderly clientele. Institutions of higher learning, faced with a declining youth population, must develop programs of learning and activity that are a source of stimulation to older people. The challenge lies in our willingness *now* to become advocates for a society that addresses the needs of our elderly, needs that surely all of us, someday, will eventually consider important.

THE PLIGHT OF THE ELDERLY

In spite of an aging population, for many, old age in America remains a tragedy. Depression, deprivation, desolation, and despair mark the lives of many elderly Americans. More than one-half of the women in this country who are 65 years or older are widowed, and more than one-third live alone. The ravages of inflation have seriously affected the economic security and vitality of many older Americans who live on fixed incomes. Approximately 3.4 million older adults live in poverty, with annual household incomes of less than $3,500 (Murphy & Florio, 1978). Over 1.2 million older people are "warehoused" in 23,000 nursing homes, at least half of which cannot pass even basic sanitation and fire-safety inspections (Butler, 1978). Discrimination among employers against the older person is widespread.

Two-thirds of the billions of dollars spent by the federal government on health care is for people over 65 (Butler, 1978). Approximately 85 percent of people over 65 have one or more chronic medical conditions such as high blood pressure, arthritis, arteriosclerosis, or heart disease (Butler, 1975). Osteoporosis, a debilitating bone disease, afflicts over 6 million Americans a year, and women make up approximately five-sixths of all victims (Smith, 1982). Medical expenditures by older persons exceed by 3.5 times those made by people under 65 (Botwinick, 1978).

The old are commonly viewed as unproductive, unemployable, inflexible, senile, and asexual. They are labeled as "over the hill," "out to pasture," "down the drain," and "old crocks" (Butler, 1975). Paradoxically, the promotion of healthful practices to preserve youth and retard aging indirectly suggests that old age is a second-rate period of life. Old age is sometimes even viewed as a second childhood. It seems that many of us have forgotten that eventual membership into this minority group is not exclusive—the only requirement is to have patience and wait our turn (Colavita, 1978).

8

The data presented here have historically reinforced a decremental perspective on aging in which aging is viewed as a period of decline. Yet, 81 percent of those over 65 years are fully ambulatory and only 4 percent are institutionalized. Although the loss of physical health, retirement, death of loved ones, and a lowered standard of living impinge on the mental health of the elderly, old age can be emotionally satisfying and a time for creativity and innovation (Butler, 1975). It would seem more appropriate to adopt a personal-growth model of aging rather than a pathological model, in which it is recognized that, in spite of loss, growing old can be a time of personal growth and fulfillment (Kalish, 1982).

PERSONAL GROWTH THROUGH PHYSICAL ACTIVITY

As early as ancient Greek times, Hippocrates noted that physical activity was beneficial to the aging process:

> Speaking generally, all parts of the body which have a function, if used in moderation and exercised in labours to which each is accustomed, become thereby healthy and well-developed, and age slowly; but if unused and left idle, they become liable to disease, defective in growth, and age quickly. (Withington, trans., 1959, pp. 339-440).

Until recently, however, the emphasis has been on moderation when discussing physical activity for the elderly. Walking has been prescribed as the universal exercise for older persons (Kamenetz, 1977). An early textbook on geriatric medicine observed: "Physical activity cannot be prolonged on account of the weakened locomotory tissues, these soon becoming tired, also on account of the increased action of the heart and lungs which cannot keep up prolonged hyperactivity without increasing their own degeneration" (Nascher, 1914, pp. 481-482). The author suggested that a walk through an unfamiliar forest path provided not only physical exercise but mental exhilaration as well. However, he cautioned us to adhere to the rule that all forms of exercise in the aged be stopped the moment fatigue sets in.

Overcoming Barriers To Participation

Lately, it has become apparent that we have underestimated the potential of older persons to derive enormous benefits from participation in vigorous physical activity. A historical emphasis on aging as a period of decline and on the frailties of the older person has promoted a sedentary life-style among the majority of older adults. Many older persons tend to overrate the benefits of light, sporadic physical activity, grossly underestimate their potential for remaining physically active, overestimate the risks associated with physical activity, and underrate their own physical abilities and capacities (Conrad, 1976).

There are examples, of course, of extraordinary athletic feats by older persons. Ruth Rothfarb ran in the New York marathon in 1981 at the age of 80 (Rosenthal, 1981). Marian McKechnie, 76, had both hips replaced after a bout with degenerative arthritis. Although she needs help climbing onto the starting block for a swimming race, she has set 16 national records for her age group in the freestyle and backstroke (Levin, 1981). Thomas Cureton, 78, sometimes called the "Father of Physical Fitness," runs, bicycles, and swims 20 miles per day. To maintain an optimum level of physical conditioning, Cureton recommended that an adult exercise a minimum of 1 hour a day until the age of 60, 2 hours a day until 70, and 3 hours a day after the age of 70 ("Father of Fitness," 1980). Russell Meyers, 77, retired professor of neurosurgery, ex-Olympian, and captain of the 1927 Brown University track team, had not run competitively again until he was 75. In the last 2 years, he has trained 6 days a week—3 days of jogging 3-4 miles and 3 days of practicing hurdles and sprints (Levin, 1981).

It can be argued that these are examples of extraordinary human beings who, in some cases, have had to overcome major physical barriers before achieving success. However, these examples also point to the potentially enormous diversity of individuals chronologically labeled as "elderly." Some older persons, crippled by degenerative disease, have extremely limited mobility. Most older Americans, however, while chronically sedentary in their life-styles, are fully ambulatory and capable of participating in a variety of progressive physical activities.

Many older adults approach physical activity with the notion that either they are too old to participate or they are too old to derive benefits from participation (Ostrow, 1980). In fact, it was not clearly documented until the late 1960's that older persons could benefit from physical training. It is now recognized that many of the known training effects associated with participation in regular programs of physical activity and exercise by younger persons can be extrapolated to the older adult—even among individuals who have been inactive for many years. Improvements in vital capacity, oxygen uptake, systolic and diastolic blood pressure, working heart rate, blood volume, percentage of body fat, and blood lactate concentrations have been reported among individuals, young or old, who engage in regular and vigorous programs of physical activity. There is also recent evidence to suggest that physical exercise, by its trophic effect on the central nervous system, may even retard age-related declines in neuromuscular efficiency and psychomotor speed (Spirduso, 1980). In addition, participation in physical activity can provide mental health benefits to the older person.

The potential physical and emotional gains that participation in physical activity can provide to older adults have been underestimated. These benefits are not contingent upon having trained vigorously in youth (deVries, 1977). Although it has been universally observed that many physical abilities appear to decline as people age, disuse or habitual inactivity rather than biological aging may be the single most important factor contributing to this decline. As deVries (1979) has aptly stated: "Ideally, physical fitness is a condition which should be achieved in youth, pursued through middle age, and never relinquished insofar as that is humanly possible" (p. 8).

Life Span and Life Expectancy

Although physical activity can contribute to personal growth through improved physical and mental health, there is no evidence that physical activity prolongs the human life span, which is our *maximum* biological age range. In fact, the human life span of 112–114 years has remained unaltered for the last three centuries (Shephard, 1978). There have been reports of individuals living to 150 years and even longer in Siberia, Tibet, and other locales. However, most of these reports have come out of remote villages where records of birth often are inaccurate (or do not exist) and, thus, investigators have frequently relied on the self-reports of those individuals whose ages are in question (Rockstein & Sussman, 1979).

The human life span appears to be mediated by both genetic and environmental factors. There appears to be a positive relationship between the longevities of parents and the corresponding longevities of their offspring (Botwinick, 1978; Shephard, 1978), although it has been difficult to isolate the role of heredity versus differences in upbringing and life-style in promoting a longer life span. Cells seem to have built-in time clocks that regulate our life span. Researchers appear to be nearer to understanding this so-called biological clock and to manipulating the mechanisms that control aging processes. For example, investigations of progeria, a rare genetic disease in which children go through the stages of development and aging at an accelerated pace (Stevens, 1981), are providing researchers with a better understanding of aging mechanisms. As Senator Alan Cranston (1981) has asked:

> Are progeria and exceptionally long-lived people simply cases of an accidentally scrambled genetic code? Is the genetic code carried out in every cell in the body, or are there master controls in the pituitary or hypothalamus of the brain or somewhere else? (p. 38)

Although the human life span has remained unchanged, the human life *expectancy*, or average age to which we might expect to live, has improved dramatically during this century. At the beginning of the century, the average life expectancy was 46 years for men and 48 years for women. By 1950, these figures increased to 66 years for men and 71 years for women (Shephard, 1978). Today, men can expect to live to 73 years

11

and women to almost 78 years. These gains are remarkable, particularly when one considers that the average life expectancy was 22 years in Caesar's day and almost 35 years in Shakespearean England (Cranston, 1981).

Rapid increments in the life expectancy of Americans can be attributed to a number of factors, including control of communicable diseases, improved health care, increased physical activity, better nutritional practices, advances in occupational safety, improved sanitary conditions, and more knowledge of the principles of hygiene and child care (Shephard, 1978). Many of these improvements, however, have resulted in a reduction of early childhood deaths rather than an improvement in the life expectancy of the mature adult (Kalish, 1982; Shephard, 1978). Although many infectious and contagious diseases have been reduced or eradicated, chronic degenerative diseases such as cancer, cerebrovascular disease, and heart disease are still leading causes of death.

GERONTOLOGY: AN EMERGING DISCIPLINE

In recent years, we have seen the rapid advancement of gerontology as a scientific discipline dedicated to understanding the elderly and aging processes. In addition, geriatrics, the system of care and treatment of the elderly, is being given greater attention by medical schools and other health-related professions. Unfortunately, as recently as 1973-74, a survey of 100 medical schools in the United States indicated that 87 percent did not offer a geriatric specialty and did not plan to expand their curricula in this area (McClusky & Altenhof, 1978).

Gerontology, by definition, is an interdisciplinary field of study. Gerontologists investigate aging processes in animals and plants as well as in human beings. Gerontology has spawned a number of subspecialties, one of the most recent of which is social gerontology, a discipline which is devoted to understanding the impact of social and cultural factors as they relate to aging.

There has been a proliferation of scientific literature on aging (see Figure 1-3). During the period 1954-74, approximately 50,000 published entries were recorded in gerontology, an amount exceeding the amount of gerontological literature of all previous years combined (Hendricks & Hendricks, 1981). In addition, Poon and Welford (1980) estimated that there was a 270 percent increase in publications related to the psychology of aging from 1968 to 1979—a span of only 11 years!

Recently, universities and other institutions of higher learning in the United States have dramatically expanded programs related to gerontology and the older adult learner. This increased interest by universities in older Americans has been fostered, in part, by a declining enrollment of students aged 18-22, by greater emphases on promoting interdisciplinary programs, and by the recognition that aging is an

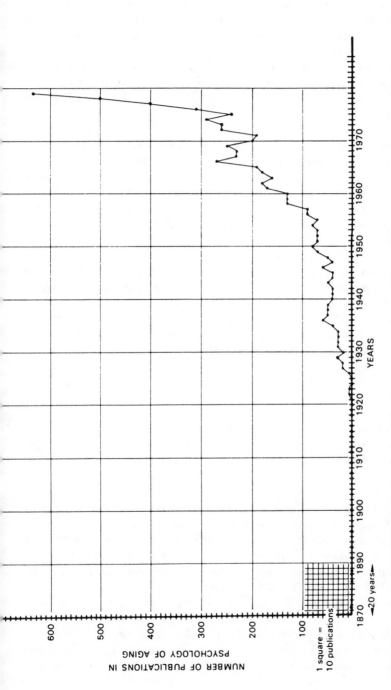

Figure 1-3. Number of psychological aging publications per year from 1880 to 1979. (From Poon, L.W., and Welford, A.T. Prologue: A historical perspective. In L.W. Poon (Ed.), *Aging in the 1980s*. Washington, D.C.: American Psychological Association, 1980, p. xiv. Copyright 1980 by the American Psychological Association. Reprinted by permission of the author and publisher.)

integral part of life-span development. Universities now offer degrees and certificates in gerontology, they have developed programs (e.g., in physical fitness) that cater to an older clientele, and they have promoted research institutes whose emphases lie in gerontology. Delegates attending the 1981 White House Conference on Aging urged the federal government to provide continued funding for educational programs that promote the social, economic, and physical well-being of older persons (Watkins, 1981).

Federal funding for service and research on aging increased dramatically during the 1970's. The National Institute on Aging, formed in 1974, was instrumental in allocating funds to support biological, behavioral, and social science research on aging; however, funding for behavioral science research areas did not keep pace with funding for the biological sciences (Poon & Welford, 1980). Recently, there has been concern that an overall reduction in governmental "bigness" will lead to a serious curtailment of federal funding in gerontology during the coming years.

Future career opportunities for individuals interested in working with older adults in a physical activity setting are promising. Retirement communities, nursing homes, YMCAs and YWCAs, and corporate industry are all in need of trained professionals in physical education and allied fields who have a sincere interest in promoting the well-being of older adults through physical activity. It is hoped that the 1980s will be remembered as the decade in which we mounted a national effort toward ensuring that all Americans remain physically active as they grow older.

SUMMARY

This chapter explored the status of being old in America and the richness of human diversity that is particularly apparent among older people. The graying of America has forced many of us to reevaluate priorities that formally have focused on a youth-oriented culture. Gerontology has emerged as an important interdisciplinary endeavor. The potential role of physical activity in enhancing life expectancy and promoting general well-being is becoming an important thrust of gerontological research. Barriers that have previously limited older adult participation in physical activity are being removed. Today, there is an increasing realization that physical activity participation must be pursued and cherished across the life cycle.

Attempts to define old age and to conveniently categorize people as old have been hampered by the enormous diversity present among older people who bring with them a history rich in life experiences. As Krauss (1980) has observed, older people are different from each other, they may be more different from each other than are younger people, and, as a group, they may be even more different from each other than they are from younger people.

Attempts to study aging effects cross-sectionally across cohorts may be suspect because of the potential confounding effects of age and culture. We must be creative in our approaches to studying older people and aging processes. Chapter 2 evaluates traditional areas of concern to the researcher in gerontology and reviews some promising research approaches and designs that may help us better understand the role of physical activity in the lives of older adults.

REFERENCES

American population growing older. *Asbury Park Press,* December 10, 1981, p. C11.

Birren, J.E., & Renner, V.J. Research on the psychology of aging: Principles and experimentation. In J.E. Birren & K.W. Schaie (Eds.), *Handbook of the psychology of aging.* New York: Van Nostrand Reinhold, 1977.

Botwinick, J. *Aging and behavior* (2nd ed.). New York: Springer, 1978.

Butler, R.N. *Why survive? Being old in America.* New York: Harper & Row, 1975.

Butler, R.N. To find the answers. In R. Gross, B. Gross, & S. Seidman (Eds.), *The new old: Struggling for decent aging.* Garden City, N.Y.: Anchor Press, 1978.

Clark, M.M. It's not all downhill! In R. Gross, B. Gross, & S. Seidman (Eds.), *The new old: Struggling for decent aging.* Garden City, N.Y.: Anchor Press, 1978.

Colavita, F.B. *Sensory changes in the elderly.* Springfield, Ill.: Charles C. Thomas, 1978.

Conrad, C.C. When you're young at heart. *Aging,* 1976, *258,* 11-13.

Cranston, A. Science slows aging. *Runner's World,* 1981, *16,* 36-40.

deVries, H.A. Physiology of physical conditioning for the elderly. In R. Harris & L.J. Frankel (Eds.), *Guide to fitness after 50.* New York: Plenum Press, 1977.

deVries, H.A. Role of exercise in aging. *American Alliance for Health, Physical Education, and Recreation News Kit on Programs for the Aging,* March 1979, 1-8.

Falk, G., Falk, V., & Tomashevich, G.V. *Aging in America and other cultures.* Saratoga, Calif.: Century Twenty One, 1981.

"Father of fitness," 78, links exercise, health. [Morgantown] *Dominion-Post,* July 29, 1980, p. 9.

Fenstermacher, G.C. Elderly sunbelt migrants. *Journal of Physical Education, Recreation, and Dance,* 1981, *52,* 57-59.

Hendricks, J., & Hendricks, C.D. *Aging in mass society: Myths and realities* (2nd ed.). Cambridge, Mass.: Winthrop, 1981.

Kalish, R.A. *Late adulthood: Perspective on human development* (2nd ed.). Monterey, Calif.: Brooks/Cole, 1982.

Kamenetz, H.L. History of exercises for the elderly. In R. Harris & L.J. Frankel (Eds.), *Guide to fitness after 50.* New York: Plenum Press, 1977.

Kenyon, G.S. A conceptual model for characterizing physical activity. *Research Quarterly,* 1968, *39,* 96-105.

Krauss, I.K. Between- and within-group comparisons in aging research. In L.W. Poon (Ed.), *Aging in the 1980s.* Washington, D.C.: American Psychological Association, 1980.

Levin, D.P. Some old Masters vault nine-foot bar—and 70 years. *Wall Street Journal,* May 28, 1981, p. 1.

McClusky, N.G., & Altenhof, J. The system makes it unhealthy to be old. In R. Gross, B. Gross, & S. Seidman (Eds.), *The new old: Struggling for decent aging.* Garden City, N.Y.: Anchor Press, 1978.

McDonald, K. 40,000 freshmen chemistry students later, Berkeley's Hildebrand celebrates 100 years. *The Chronicle of Higher Education,* November 25, 1981, p. 2.

16

Murphy, J., & Florio, C. Older Americans: Facts and potential. In R. Gross, B. Gross, & S. Seidman (Eds.), *The new old: Struggling for decent aging.* Garden City, N.Y.: Anchor Press, 1978.

Nascher, I.L. *Geriatrics: The diseases of old age and their treatment.* Philadelphia: P. Blakiston's & Son, 1914.

Neugarten, B.L. The future and the young-old. *The Gerontologist,* 1975, *15* (1., Pt. 2), 4-9.

Now, the revolt of the old. *Time,* October 10, 1977, pp. 18-28.

Ostrow, A.C. Physical activity as it relates to the health of the aged. In N. Datan & N. Lohmann (Eds.), *Transitions of aging.* New York: Academic Press, 1980.

Poon, L.W., & Welford, A.T. Prologue: A historical perspective. In L.W. Poon (Ed.), *Aging in the 1980s.* Washington, D.C.: American Psychological Association, 1980.

Rockstein, M., & Sussman, M. *Biology of aging.* Belmont, Calif.: Wadsworth, 1979.

Rosenthal, B. Salazar seeking world mark in Sunday's NYC marathon. [Morgantown] *Dominion-Post,* October 24, 1981, p. 2B.

Shephard, R.J. *Physical activity and aging.* Chicago: Year Book Medical Publishers, 1978.

Smith, S. Learn how to take care and take charge. [Morgantown] *Dominion-Post,* September 26, 1982, p. 1-E.

Spirduso, W.W. Physical fitness, aging, and psychomotor speed: A review. *Journal of Gerontology,* 1980, *35,* 850-865.

Stevens, C. Little old boys meet, plan visit with third progeria victim. [Morgantown] *Dominion-Post,* December 1, 1981, p. 6-B.

U.S. Bureau of the Census. *Age, sex, race, and Spanish origin of the population by regions, divisions, and states: 1980* (Supplementary Report PC80-S1-1). Washington, D.C.: U.S. Department of Commerce, May 1981.

Watkins, B.T. A "full range of educational programs" for the aging. *The Chronicle of Higher Education,* December 9, 1981, p. 22.

Withington, E.T. (trans.). *Hippocrates* (Vol. 3). Cambridge, Mass.: Harvard University Press, 1959.

17

2

The Research Process

In recent years, exercise programs and other programs of physical activity for the elderly have emerged throughout the United States. These programs, while admirable in their goals, have lacked adequate scientific information on how best to meet the physical activity needs of the older adult. For example, it is not uncommon for some physical activity programs to promote a task in which a large group of older persons stand in a circle and use a large sheet to propel a ball through the air. Intuitively, it would seem that this task was designed to promote social interaction and, possibly, gross motor coordination. Unfortunately, the expected outcomes of this task may be based more on wishful thinking than carefully evaluated scientific evidence.

Research based on the scientific method permits us to gather systematically information that ultimately will enable us to explain, predict, and modify the impact of aging on motor skill acquisition and performance. By adhering to appropriate sampling procedures and research designs, by systematically ruling out alternative explanations, and by employing measurement tools that have been carefully validated to permit empirical assessment, we can logically test hypotheses that form the foundation for theory development and program practice.

There are many questions that remain unresolved with respect to the impact of physical activity on the older adult and aging processes. For example, what forms of physical activity are most effective in reducing anxiety and depression among older adults? What is the optimal exercise training regimen for delaying age-related declines in central nervous system processing or in preventing the onset of osteoporosis among postmenopausal women? How can we modify societal role expectations that dictate a more sedentary life-style among older Americans?

In our rush to set up programs of physical activity for older persons, we must insist on the development of a concomitant knowledge base upon which the rationale and methodologies of these programs are founded. Programmatic decisions must be based on more than just sound intuitive thinking, or experiential judgment, to avoid the risk of "turning off" our older citizenry from participating in physical activity. Toward this end, it is vital to understand the research process as it directly relates to studying aging and the older adult involved in physical activity.

MAJOR RESEARCH QUESTIONS

Several important questions arise when we examine the research literature on physical activity and the older adult. These questions relate to the true effects of aging versus observed age differences, whether a product-oriented or process-oriented approach is used, and the usefulness of laboratory and "real-world" studies.

Aging or Age Differences?

Suppose the novice investigator is interested in determining if individuals develop more negative attitudes toward physical activity participation with advancing age. To answer this question, a commonly employed research strategy would be for this investigator to administer to randomly selected groups of subjects who vary in chronological age a carefully validated "Attitudes Toward Physical Activity Participation" scale. A hypothetically derived data set is graphically represented in Figure 2-1, in which a lower attitude score is indicative of a more negative attitude toward physical activity participation. Based on a statistical analysis of these data, the naive investigator might erroneously conclude that people generally develop more negative attitudes toward participating in physical activity because they advance in age.

Unfortunately, this investigator has failed to tease out the potential confounding effects of cohort or cultural differences in his effort to understand the impact of aging on attitude formation and change. It can easily be argued that these observed age differences in attitude are representative of a number of cultural factors unique to each cohort randomly sampled. For example, although the 60–69 age group appears to have the most negative attitude toward physical activity participation (Figure 2-1), this may be due to a general unavailability of physical education programs and opportunities when they were younger, factors that were eventually ameliorated for the younger age groups studied. Thus, while this research design permits us to *describe* age differences, difficulties develop when trying to *explain* that these observed age differences are indicative of the impact of aging on attitude change. The age differences observed may simply be differences among cohorts. As we shall see shortly, this is a common problem facing researchers who employ a cross-sectional research design to studying aging processes.

Product-oriented or Process-oriented Approach?

In examining the aging literature in relation to physical activity, it will become apparent that two general approaches have been taken in studying motor skills: the product-oriented approach and the process-oriented approach (Schmidt, 1982). The product-oriented approach to studying physical activity and movement behavior focuses on the outcomes of human performance. The goal of this scientific orientation

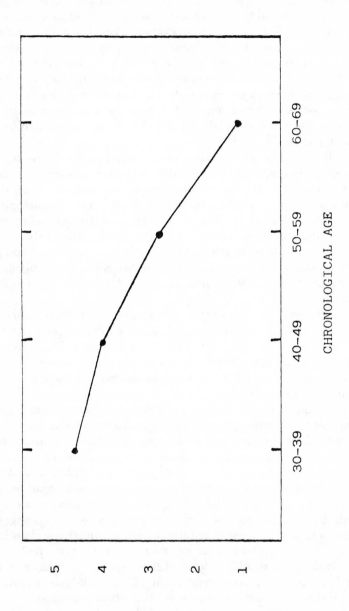

Figure 2-1. Attitudes toward physical activity participation among four cohorts (hypothetical data).

in the study of human movement is, generally, to investigate various independent variables as they affect observed motor performance scores on a variety of tasks. In a typical experiment, the effects of psychological stress on motor performance might be examined based on a computation of error or speed scores. From the results of this experiment, one might infer that psychological stress inhibits motor performance based on observed increases in error scores or decrements in speed. However, there is little systematic effort to explain the outcome (or product). In other words, the product-oriented approach fails to consider the underlying mechanisms and processes by which psychological stress ultimately leads to performance inhibition.

The bulk of the research literature on aging and physical activity has been product oriented. Data from Hodgkins (1963) nicely illustrate this point (see Figure 2-2). In this cross-sectional study, Hodgkins examined reaction time (RT) and movement time (MT) in relation to chronological age and gender. A total of 930 men, women, and children, who were categorized into seven age cohorts (e.g., first grade and elderly), were tested. They were asked to release a telegraph key with their hand in response to a randomly presented light stimulus (RT) and to move their arm horizontally as rapidly as possible (MT) to a terminating rod 23½ inches away.

As can be seen in Figure 2-2, the outcomes of these subjects' performances are expressed in units of time. These data suggest that RT and MT become substantially slower after early adulthood. Certainly our next question (if we have confidence that these data are not confounded by variables other than age effects) should address *why* there are these apparent age decrements.

Recently, the process-oriented approach has become the more dominant route in studying motor learning and control (Schmidt, 1982). This approach focuses on the underlying processes accounting for movement rather than on the terminal outcomes of movement. The processes related to aging and movement are essentially physical and/or biochemical changes observed at the cellular, tissue, and organ levels. Motor behavior researchers who have adopted the process-oriented approach have been concerned with such issues as the coding of information in memory, neurological mechanisms underlying attention during movement, and the existence of motor programs. Tasks are specifically designed to address some of these issues, and measurement approaches, such as electromyographic (EMG) analysis, examine neurological mechanisms responsible for movement execution.

The process-oriented approach is beginning to have an impact on motor skills and aging research. For example, a popular way of conceptualizing human movement is based on an information-processing model. Simply put, this model assumes that the individual

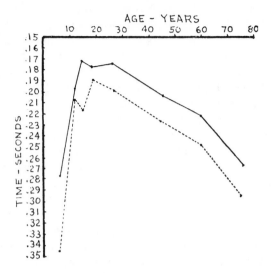

Figure 2-2. Cross-sectional data on differences in RT (dashed line) and MT (solid line) as a function of chronological age. (From Hodgkins, J. Reaction time and speed of movement in males and females of various ages. *Research Quarterly*, 1963, *34*, 340. Reprinted by permission of the American Alliance for Health, Physical Education, Recreation, and Dance, 1900 Association Drive, Reston, VA 22091.)

actively selects, processes, and stores information vital to movement performance. Birren, Woods, and Williams (1980) summarized the results of a number of investigations that have adopted an information-processing model in an effort to understand behavioral slowing in relation to advancing age.

I will have more to say about information processing and aging effects in Chapter 3. It is sufficient to note, at this point, that product-oriented research on aging and motor skills must be complemented by a process-oriented approach if we are to eventually understand the impact of aging on skillful performance. A natural outgrowth of combining these two approaches is theory development, which ultimately will pave the way toward a better understanding of aging and physical activity.

The Laboratory or the Real World?

The Hodgkins (1963) study on RT and MT is typical of the design of many studies on behavioral slowing in relation to aging. A study of this nature lends itself to the possibility that variables other than chronological age may be confounded in this design. Thus, a major objective of the scientific method is to generate data that provide unambiguous answers to a given research problem (Baltes, Reese, & Nesselroade, 1977). By minimizing extraneous variables, we help ensure the *internal validity* of our design, that is, our ability to rule out alternative explanations.

Scientists often select the laboratory for the investigation of developmental research problems because of the greater opportunity to test subjects in a controlled environment. Thus, Hodgkins (1963) tested subjects in a laboratory-type environment on an apparatus specifically designed to measure RT and MT. Ultimately, however, the goal of the developmentalist is to explain, predict, and perhaps modify "naturally" occurring behaviors (Baltes et al., 1977). The question that needs to be raised in regard to the Hodgkins study, as well as other laboratory studies of this nature, is, Can we generalize these findings to the realm of physical activity?

The *external validity* of a research design addresses the question of the extent to which our results are generalizable to other populations, settings, treatment variables, and measurement variables. In carrying out a research project, scientists often try to achieve an optimum "internal validity–external validity balance"; that is, although they recognize the need for carefully controlled projects to ensure interpretable results, they also recognize that the trade-off on control is sometimes an inability to project their findings to the real world. As Schmidt (1982) has humorously suggested, however, "the outside world is, at best, an inexact and incomplete approximation to the real world of the laboratory" (p. 30). In other words, there may be some question about where "reality" really is.

I believe that the important question with regard to physical activity is not whether laboratory or real world research is more valid but, rather, under what circumstances the gains from controlled laboratory research (e.g., in terms of theory development) are worth their potential limited applicability to understanding physical activity. Similarly, the long-term costs, imprecision, and possible specificity of applied (real-world) research must be carefully weighed, a priori.

Issues of external validity are complex, particularly in developmental research. Besides the traditional mechanistic concerns expressed by Campbell and Stanley (1963) in their classical treatment of research design and external validity, there are potentially different qualitative principles introduced by studying people at different ages and developmental levels (Baltes et al., 1977). After all, the domain of observations that developmentalists ultimately seek to make a statement on is not static.

In reviewing research reported in this book, the reader should ask to what extent this information is truly applicable to understanding the impact physical activity has on the older adult. Often, the researcher has spent considerably more time regulating potential threats to internal validity than systematically planning for the potential generalizability of his/her results. Although it is quantitatively difficult to evaluate or ensure external validity, researchers must be more attentive to and creative in the ways they attempt to maximize the external validity of their designs if their data are to have bearing on understanding physical activity and the older adult.

RESEARCH DESIGNS

A major objective of research design is to provide the most efficient and effective means of generating unambiguous answers to a set of research problems. There is probably no ideal research design for answering a given research problem; one has to weigh the potential threats to internal validity, the cost-effectiveness, feasibility, and efficiency of the design, and the merits of the research design in terms of generalization.

Cross-sectional Design

The research design employed by Hodgkins (1963) to study RT and MT, in which two or more age groups are studied in a single period of time, is usually referred to as a cross-sectional design. It has been the most commonly employed research design for studying age differences in the realm of physical activity and inferring reasons for any age differences derived. The cross-sectional design often appears to be the logical choice for investigating a developmental research problem, because it permits the rapid investigation of the problem using a large number of subjects who often can conveniently be group tested in one setting at minimal cost to the investigator. However, as Botwinick (1978) has aptly stated "an observed age difference today may not be seen tomorrow" (p. 365).

As stated earlier, we must be extremely cautious when attempting to attribute age effects to observed age differences, because these aging effects may be confounded by culturally based cohort differences. Furthermore, selective survival rates may hopelessly confound interpretation of any observed age differences (Baltes et al., 1977). In studying attitudes toward physical activity participation, we could refine our design (and thus achieve some control) by selecting age groups that have been matched on those variables that we feel may also account for any observed age differences. For example, we could control for previous physical education opportunities by matching subjects in each age group who self-report (based on questionnaire responses) less than or more than 2 years of required physical education classes in high school. However, there may be many variables worthy of subject matching, and adequate matching is difficult to achieve across different cohorts. In addition, the matching process denies us some of the benefits gained from random subject selection.

The cross-sectional research design will probably continue to remain popular in the developmental literature. This design permits us, to some extent, to identify interindividual differences and is certainly of value in pilot research when examining possible age differences in the realm of physical activity. However, we must be extremely sensitive to the potential confounding effects of age and culture when this design is used to explain rather than describe age-related phenomena.

Longitudinal Design

Another research design employed in the developmental literature is the longitudinal design, in which a particular cohort is repeatedly assessed across time, usually for a duration of at least several years. At first glance, this design would seem to permit us to explain aging effects better than the cross-sectional approach. However, Botwinick (1978) cautions us that any observed maturational changes could also be confounded by concomitant cultural changes. This is particularly apparent in a long-term longitudinal study.

For example, let us speculate on the results we might obtain if we were to assess repeatedly a cohort born in the period 1920–29 on their attitudes toward physical activity participation. We might observe increasingly negative attitudes as we analyze their scores during the late 1960's and early 1970's. To our surprise, however, these attitude scores could stabilize (or even become more positive) as we continue to study this cohort during the remainder of the 1970's. Have maturational aging effects caused this reversal, or has America's sudden enchantment with physical fitness during the late 1970's affected the attitude scores of this cohort? This is an example of what might be labeled the "cultural-maturational paradox."

The longitudinal design permits a more accurate description of intraindividual variation than the cross-sectional approach, although Shephard (1978) cautions us that many physiological variables may require 15 or even 20 years of repeated testing to define adequately the rate of aging. Longitudinal studies, therefore, require large numbers of subjects and may turn out to be extremely costly and time consuming. The external validity of the longitudinal study may be limited, at best, to extrapolations to the population from which the cohort has been drawn. Subject attrition (because of boredom, moving, death, and other factors) must be carefully controlled and/or evaluated when generalizations are to be made to other members of the cohort population. In addition, the repeated assessment of individuals introduces possible subject practice effects and changes in subject motivation, interest, and experimenter expectations, all of which may distort the results of the investigation. Furthermore, scientific advances may make some instrumentation obsolete. The investigator is then faced with the dilemma of adding new instrumentation at the risk of distorting the validity of results previously obtained.

Alterations can be made in the design of a longitudinal study to control for some of these problems, and systematic retrieval procedures can be developed to reduce the impact of subject attrition. An excellent discussion of some of these methods is presented by Baltes, Reese, and Nesselroade (1977) and Botwinick (1978). It is sufficient to indicate here that an investigator interested in conducting a longitudinal study must determine initially if the problem under consideration warrants the longitudinal method. Commitment to a longitudinal study requires great patience, sacrifice, discipline, and an understanding that, at best, the payoff remains far down the road.

Sequential Designs

Before concluding a discussion of research designs, I would be remiss if I did not consider the potential use of sequential designs in the study of physical activity and aging. In an article that has been of major significance in improving developmental research designs, Schaie (1965) proposed a tri-factor developmental model of aging. This model attempts to account for the interactions of three major factors or sources of variation important to developmental change: maturation (aging), cohort, and time of measurement, Table 2-1 illustrates these three factors.

As can be seen in this table, the cross-sectional design (four cohorts who vary in age tested at one point in time) is illustrated diagonally and the

Table 2-1

Sequential Strategies

Cohort	Chronological age				
	30	40	50	60	
1930	1930	1940	1950	1960	→ Cross-sectional sequences
1940	1940	1950	1960	1970	
1950	1950	1960	1970	1980	→ Longitudinal sequences
1960	1960	1970	1980	1990	

Note. Adapted from *Life-span developmental psychology: Introduction to research methods,* by P.B. Baltes, H.W. Reese, and J.R. Nesselroade. Copyright © 1977 by Wadsworth Publishing Company, Inc. Reprinted by permission of the publisher, Brooks/Cole Publishing Company, Monterey, California.

27

longitudinal design (one cohort tested at different ages, four points in time) is illustrated horizontally. In addition, a vertical examination of the table illustrates a potential *time-lag* design in which people of the same age from different cohorts are tested at different points in time. The cross-sectional design confounds age x cohort differences, the longitudinal design confounds age x time-of-measurement differences, and the time-lag design confounds cohort x time-of-measurement differences. Thus, each design is confounded by two sources of variation.

Sequential designs have been proposed as a means of disentangling these three interacting factors and better accounting for intraindividual developmental change (Baltes et al., 1977; Botwinick, 1978). Baltes and co-workers (1977) refer to *cross-sectional sequences* as a research strategy in which independent observations are obtained across all cohort levels and all age levels. For example, the 1950 and 1960 testings of the 1940 cohort (Table 2-1) would be done using different random samples of the 1940 cohort. This is really an extension of the cross-sectional design in that more than one time of measurement is obtained. In *longitudinal sequences* (Table 2-1), repeated assessments are made within all cohorts. For example, a sample of subjects from the 1950 cohort is tested in 1950 and again in 1960; a sample is also selected from the 1960 cohort and these persons are tested in 1960 and 1970.

Baltes and co-workers (1977) maintained that cross-sectional sequences and longitudinal sequences, when used simultaneously, can help provide accurate descriptions of intraindividual and interindividual developmental changes. Sequential designs enable us to tease out age changes from cohort changes. However, sequential designs are of limited explanatory value in understanding developmental change. They are difficult designs to execute and costly to carry out. As we explore the literature on physical activity and aging, it will become apparent that this literature is primarily based on the use of the cross-sectional research design. Little, if any, attempt has been made to introduce sequential designs as a viable alternative to studying physical activity and its impact on the older adult.

SAMPLING OLDER PEOPLE

In studying older people, we are faced with several interesting sampling considerations. Older persons bring with them a history rich in life experiences. Unfortunately (for the research investigator), these experiences contribute to the enormous heterogeneity observed within older people and between older people and younger people. This sometimes prevents the researcher from nicely packaging the results obtained on older people into classical statistical models. Thus, statisticians often label within-subject variability as error when attempting to study differences between groups.

The problem of teasing out age changes from cultural differences when comparing different cohorts is further confounded by the fact that older people who volunteer to participate in physical activity research studies may not be representative of older people in general. These people are generally healthier and have better functional mobility. In addition, it is well known (e.g., Rosenthal & Rosnow, 1969) that volunteers often bring with them a unique set of personality characteristics that may limit the external validity (generalizability) of the obtained results.

Another problem in sampling is that volunteerism seems to be inversely correlated to chronological age (Shephard, 1978). In a study conducted a few years ago (Ostrow, 1980), I sought to establish the construct validity of a conceptual model characterizing attitudes older people held toward participating in physical activity. Of the 800 questionnaires distributed to older adults residing in a retirement community in New Jersey, only 62 usable questionnaires (or 8 percent) were returned. In an effort to obtain adequate samples of older people, some investigators have, therefore, relied heavily on captive audiences.

The researcher conducting a longitudinal study in the area of physical activity and aging is also faced with the dilemma of differential subject attrition. As Botwinick (1978) has noted, healthier older people are more likely to survive during long-term study. This poses a problem, particularly to researchers studying physical activity. Selective dropout rates tend to distort the results obtained and may limit the generalizability of the findings. For example, in a study examining the long-term physical and mental health benefits of a physical exercise program, we might erroneously conclude that the exercise program produced beneficial change, when, in fact, the retention of only very healthy older people in the study promoted these distorted results.

As an alternative strategy to the group research design, it is surprising that few investigators have explored the feasibility and potentiality of the single-subject design (e.g., Hersen & Barlow, 1976). This design, in which one or several subjects are selected for intensive study, would seem particularly appropriate for research (or at least pilot research) on older people and physical activity. Many of the sampling problems previously identified are eliminated. This design allows for a more holistic and intensive examination of older people. Of course, the external population validity of the results may be limited initially to only those people studied. Nevertheless, many older people (and younger people) are reluctant to be treated as part of a group statistic. The single-subject study may provide a more personal approach that could, in turn, increase the probability of greater older adult participation in a long-term study on physical activity and aging.

MEASURING OLDER PEOPLE

The confining of older adults to the human performance laboratory when studying the complex interactions of movement execution and age poses some unique measurement problems for the investigator. As I will document further in Chapter 3, older adults approach the requirements of a motor task with greater cautiousness. They have lower performance expectations than young people (Gallagher, Thompson, & Levy, 1980). Older adults are increasingly susceptible to fatigue, particularly if the task is strenuous or if the trials are long in duration. They may be less motivated or more fearful of completing the performance requirements of a task. These factors, plus increasing performance variability that is commonly observed with advancing age, may lead to lower reliability estimations for a given task. Furthermore, sensory declines with advancing age (e.g., in audition and visual acuity) may distort performance comparisons across age. An experiment conducted in a poorly illuminated environment makes it particularly difficult to obtain accurate data among older people. The investigator who fails to clearly articulate and repeat slowly pretask instructions may be setting up the older person for poorer performance scores.

Concerns of measurement in relation to physical activity extend beyond obtaining error-reduced performance data in the laboratory. Much of the research examining the impact of exercise and other forms of physical activity on the mental health of the older adult have relied on self-report paper-and-pencil tests of personality. There are very few personality tests available that are specifically standardized for use by the older adult. Normative data on older adults are almost nonexistent for these personality tests. Frequently, the directions and content of personality tests are ambiguous or inappropriate for older populations (Gallagher et al., 1980). These factors, coupled with test-taking problems and the increasing variability of older people when responding, make many personality tests of questionable reliability and validity when applied to older populations (Labouvie, 1980).

We cannot assume that obtained personality test score differences across age indicate that these age groups are, in fact, different on the personality characteristics being assessed. It is also possible that the scores are not directly comparable across age groups because the items have different meanings for each age group (Baltes et al., 1977; Labouvie, 1980). For example, a test item that asks a respondent if he/she is willing to toil long hours to gain a berth on the Olympic team may not be a meaningful test item to assess achievement motivation among all age groups under investigation.

When examining the intercorrelations of various measures across several age groups we cannot be sure that the units of measurement are equal or invariant across age (Baltes et al., 1977; Labouvie, 1980).

Furthermore, Cunningham's (1978) methodological overview of comparative factor analysis makes it clear that if the standard deviations of various measures are different across different age groups, then a comparison of the factors extracted from the correlation matrices within each age group may be distorted because of a different metric being imposed on each matrix. For example, differences observed in the psychomotor ability factor structures of various age groups may be an artifact of the increasing response variability of the older age groups. Cunningham outlined several statistical procedures that can be used to alleviate this problem.

There is an obvious need to develop measures of human behavior and physical performance that are germane to the older adult. One approach might be the greater employment of systematic behavioral observation techniques in a naturalistic physical activity environment. This approach may overcome some of the measurement problems inherent in the contrived psychological testing of older adults.

DEVELOPMENTAL RESEARCH STRATEGIES: THE EXAMPLE OF LIFE EXPECTANCY

A most obvious and persistent finding in life expectancy research is the importance of good health and physical functioning (Botwinick, 1978). Intuitively, therefore, it would seem logical to postulate that physical activity can increase our life expectancy through its positive effect on physical and mental health. Active people tend to be less liable to obesity or diabetes, have reduced blood lipids, are more health conscious, sleep more regularly, and are better able to cope with stress (Shephard, 1978). However, it has been difficult to demonstrate empirically that physical activity does, in fact, directly affect human life expectancy.

In this section, I will outline several research strategies that have been adopted to answer the question of whether physical activity prolongs human life expectancy. This overview will illustrate some of the problems inherent in epidemiologic research that are also apparent in most forms of developmental investigation. In addition, an overview of some of the research findings on this question will be presented.

Milvy, Forbes, and Brown (1977) suggested that it has been difficult to determine the effect of participation in physical activity on life expectancy because most of the research has been correlational rather than causal in focus and design. They outlined four research strategies that have been used to determine the effect of physical activity on the life expectancy, as well as in other areas of epidemiologic study: the field (or "snapshot") study, the prospective study, the retrospective (case-control) study, and the clinical trial study.

The *field study* is a cross-sectional research design in which "one-shot" comparisons on a dependent variable(s) are made within a population or between populations. For example, an investigator might be interested in determining if the number of deaths (dependent variable) in a given week was related to whether one was physically active or not physically active (the so-called independent variable or classification variable) at the time of death. This is a very weak research strategy if one is interested in determining the effect of physical activity on life expectancy; not only must one clearly define the concept of "being physically active," but many other variables that could also affect life expectancy (such as the age and/or physical health of the individual) must be carefully controlled.

In a *prospective study*, the postulated cause(s) of the dependent variable (such as number of deaths) is studied in a sample(s) of individuals over time. For example, individuals who decided to become physically active could be compared over time to those individuals who never became physically active to see if there are eventual differences in the time and causes of death between the two groups.

It may seem that this approach gives us better insight into the effects of physical activity on life expectancy. However, problems of subject self-selection to the groups being compared and the difficulty of controlling the subsequent life events of these individuals make it hazardous to establish causal relationships using this design. For example, those individuals who chose to become physically active may have had family histories of greater longevity and prosperity. In addition, extensive costs and problems of measurement over time using the longitudinal method make this approach difficult to carry out.

In a *retrospective study*, individuals in whom the dependent variable (e.g., deceased) is observed are carefully matched (e.g., on age, socioeconomic status, or presence of heart disease) to individuals in whom the dependent variable is not observed (i.e., still alive). The previous histories of the subjects are carefully examined to determine if the so-called independent variable (in this case, physical activity) occurred with greater frequency and intensity in one of the groups. Perhaps an illustration of a recent retrospective study would be beneficial.

Rose and Cohen (1977) conducted a retrospective analysis of 500 white male deaths that occurred in Boston in 1965 to determine the effects of physical activity on life expectancy. These deaths occurred after the age of 50 and were not due to suicide, homicide, or accident. The age at death was distributed into four equal age ranges—50–59, 60–69, 70–79, and 80 and over—and there was an equal number of subjects ($N = 125$) in each group. The investigators interviewed the wives and children of these deceased individuals. Physical activity was operationally defined in terms of both on-the-job and off-the-job activity. They examined 198 variables, in addition to physical activity, to assess their relative contributions to life expectancy, and they found that physical activity (off the job) was a better predictor of life expectancy than over two-thirds of the variables they considered. Interestingly, however, as can be seen from the stepwise multiple regression analysis conducted (Table 2-2), cigarette-smoking frequency, appearing youthful, number of illnesses, and five other variables were more important predictors of life expectancy than physical activity.

Table 2-2

Best Predictors of Age at Death by Stepwise
Multiple Regression Analysis

Step	Predictor	Education controlled r^2 Change (%)	r^a	Step	Education not controlled r^2 Change (%)	r^a
1	Younger age appearance ≥ 40	20.2	0.47	2	9.8	0.46
2	Illness mean	9.9	-0.46	1	22.2	-0.47
3	Smoking < 40	4.3	-0.29	>10		
4	Mother's age at death	1.8	0.18	7	1.4	0.16
5	Sense of humor	1.9	-0.09*	5	2.0	-0.11†
6	Urban vs. rural residence	1.4	0.24	8	1.1	0.28
7	Intelligence	1.2	0.20	>10		
8	Worried	1.1	-0.28	6	1.4	-0.30
9	Off-job activity 40-49	0.8	0.23	9	1.1	0.20
10	Off-job activity < 20	1.6	-0.03 (NS)	10	1.7	-0.08*
>10	Smoking ≥ 40			3	4.3	-0.28
>10	Foreign vs. native born			4	2.9	-0.27
Total r^2		44.2			47.9	

Note. Adapted from "Relative Importance of Physical Activity for Longevity" by C.L. Rose and M.L. Cohen, *Annals of the New York Academy of Sciences*, 1977, *301*, 671–697. Copyright © 1977 by the New York Academy of Sciences. Reprinted by permission.

^{a}Unmarked r values are significant at the 0.01 level.
* Indicates significance at the 0.05 level.
† Indicates significance at the 0.01 level.

The Rose and Cohen study nicely illustrates the retrospective method. However, this approach still is limited in terms of identifying causal relationships. Subject self-selection to the groups and on the variables being examined is still a problem, and it is difficult to know the extent to which physical activity was sustained by these subjects during their life course. Furthermore, it is often difficult to match subjects adequately on many potentially interacting variables.

The *clinical trial study* is an example of the "true" experimental design in which subjects are randomly selected and randomly assigned to intervention(s) or independent variable(s) and the effect of these interventions or independent variables is observed on the dependent variable(s). For example, individuals randomly selected from a given population could be randomly assigned to participate in a physical activity program, a ceramic program, or no program at all, and the effects of both interventions could be observed on the frequency of deaths (dependent variable) over time. Although the clinical trial study would seem to be the most controlled and direct approach to studying the effects of physical activity on life expectancy, Montoye (1975) warns us that the number of individuals required to ensure adequate generalization and to minimize the potential effects of mortality (i.e., subject dropout) could approach 36,000 individuals if the experiment was carried out longitudinally for 5 years.

Physical activity is (or could be) beneficial to most Americans, but it has been difficult to link directly physical activity to life expectancy. Almost all the research literature in this area has been correlational rather than causal in design. The life expectancies of athletes to nonathletes have been compared, but, with the possible exception of cross-country skiers (Karvonen, Klemola, Virkajarvi, & Kekkonen, 1974) and college oarsmen (Prout, 1972), there is little evidence to suggest that athletes live longer than the general population.

Olson, Teitelbaum, Van Huss, and Montoye (1977) found that 628 athletes and 563 nonathletes from Michigan State University who had dates of birth ranging from 1855 to 1919 did not differ in their mean ages at death (see Table 2-3). Years of sport participation did not materially affect the life expectancy of these individuals, a result supported by Polednak (1972) in an assessment of the mean age at death of 681 former Harvard College athletes. Largey (1972) reported that the life expectancies of athletes appeared to be functionally related to the sports in which they had participated, with football players having the shortest life expectancy (57.4 years) and track and field athletes the longest (71.3 years). Karvonen and co-workers (1974) found that the mean age at death of Finnish male cross-country skiers exceeded by 4–5 years the mean age at death of the general male population, although it should be noted that Finland's adult mortality rate is high, particularly for men. Similarly, Prout (1972) found that 172 oarsmen at Harvard and Yale lived longer than random samples of college nonoarsmen from these institutions. In contrast, Ogawa (1979) reported that Japanese sumo wrestlers lived 7.8 years less than the general Japanese population!

The majority of these investigations might be classified as field studies. Many variables other than being an athlete, such as persistence in physical activity throughout life, frequency of cigarette smoking, and incidence of cardiac disease, may also influence mortality and need to be carefully controlled. Definitions of athlete are not clear, and different

Table 2-3

A Comparison of the Mean Age at Death of Athletes vs. Nonathletes

| | *Cohort (date of birth)* | | |
	1855–84	1885–99	1900–19
Athletes			
N	77	57	46
mean age	73.19	67.14	50.09
Nonathletes			
N	57	56	27
mean age	76.35	65.43	50.04

Note. The lower mean age at death of the two most recent cohorts was expected since many of the subjects in these two cohorts are still living. Adapted from "Years of Sports Participation and Mortality in College Athletes" by H.W. Olson, H. Teitelbaum, W.D. Van Huss, and H.J. Montoye, *Journal of Sports Medicine and Physical Fitness,* 1977, *17,* 321-326. Copyright © 1977 by Edizioni Minerva Medica. Reprinted by permission.

physical activities may affect different subpopulations at different points in the life span (Milvy et al., 1977).

In conclusion, there is little direct evidence, based on these research designs, to state definitively that physical activity alone affects the human life expectancy. Illustrative of this point are the inhabitants of the Abkhasia region of Soviet Georgia. These mountain people are models of fitness in old age—they work in their gardens, ride horseback, and bathe in icy streams well into their 80's. However, their greater life expectancy and physical vigor can be attributed not only to exercise, but also to diet, the right genes, a sense of being needed, and the respect of the community ("No telling," 1977). Thus, as deVries (1974) has aptly indicated, physical activity (by itself) may not add years to our lives, but it can certainly help add life to our remaining years.

SUMMARY

This chapter examined the research process, with special attention directed toward those research issues most germane to studying the role of physical activity in the lives of older adults. In reading subsequent chapters, it is important to distinguish between those empirical studies that deal with the effects of physical activity on aging and those studies that really describe age differences in response to physical activity participation. The bulk of research studies that we will review are of the snapshot variety and employ the cross-sectional design. Thus, these studies have really focused on age differences rather than on aging effects.

The strengths and weaknesses of the cross-sectional research design, the longitudinal design, and sequential designs were outlined in this chapter. I am not aware of any investigations on the older adult and physical activity that have utilized sequential strategies. Perhaps the complexities and costs involved have made this approach less appealing for researchers. The single-subject experimental paradigm, while not prominent in the research literature, seems particularly suited for initial research on physical activity and the older adult, because it offers a more personal and control-effective approach toward subject evaluation.

The unique concerns of sampling and measuring older people were also reviewed in this chapter. Strategies need to be developed to ensure greater participation by older adults in research on physical activity; to minimize the selective attrition of subjects, particularly in long-term study; and to ensure measurement equivalence among test batteries employed when studying physical activity and the older adult.

I concluded this chapter by illustrating the application of research design to the question of whether physical activity prolongs human life expectancy. It became clear that the dominant use of correlation designs precluded a definitive statement that physical activity does, in fact, affect the human life expectancy.

The research process not only ensures that knowledge regarding physical activity and the older adult is systematically developed, but concomitantly, enables program leaders to evolve programs of physical activity for the older adult that go beyond sound intuitive or experiential judgment. The mutual evolution of research-based knowledge and program practice is vital if our efforts toward promoting a more physically active older citizenry are to be viewed as credible and worthwhile.

REFERENCES

Baltes, P.B., Reese, H.W., & Nesselroade, J.R. *Life-span developmental psychology: Introduction to research methods.* Monterey, Calif.: Brooks/Cole, 1977.

Birren, J.E., Woods, A.M., & Williams, M.V. Behavioral slowing with age: Causes, organization, and consequences. In L.W. Poon (Ed.), *Aging in the 1980s.* Washington, D.C.: American Psychological Association, 1980.

Botwinick, J. *Aging and behavior* (2nd ed.). New York: Springer, 1978.

Campbell, D.T., & Stanley, J.C. Experimental and quasi-experimental designs for research on teaching. In N.L. Gage (Ed.), *Handbook of research on teaching.* Chicago: Rand McNally, 1963.

Cunningham, W.R. Principles for identifying structural differences. *Journal of Gerontology,* 1978, *33,* 82–86.

deVries, H.A. *Vigor regained.* Englewood Cliffs, N.J.: Prentice-Hall, 1974.

Gallagher, D., Thompson, L.W., & Levy, S.M. Clinical psychological assessment of older adults. In L.W. Poon (Ed.), *Aging in the 1980s.* Washington, D.C.: American Psychological Association, 1980.

Hersen, M., & Barlow, D.H. *Single case experimental designs: Strategies for studying behavior change.* New York: Pergamon Press, 1976.

Hodgkins, J. Reaction time and speed of movement in males and females of various ages. *Research Quarterly,* 1963, *34,* 335–343.

Karvonen, M.J., Klemola, H., Virkajarvi, J., & Kekkonen, A. Longevity of endurance skiers. *Medicine and Science in Sports,* 1974, *6,* 49–51.

Labouvie, E.W. Identity versus equivalence of psychological measures and constructs. In L.W. Poon (Ed.), *Aging in the 1980s.* Washington, D.C.: American Psychological Association, 1980.

Largey, G. Athletic activity and longevity. *Lancet,* 1972, *2*(7771), 286.

Milvy, P., Forbes, W.F., & Brown, K.S. A critical review of epidemiological studies of physical activity. *Annals of the New York Academy of Sciences,* 1977, *301,* 519–549.

Montoye, H.J. *Physical activity and health: An epidemiologic study of an entire community.* Englewood Cliffs, N.J.: Prentice-Hall, 1975.

No telling how old is old. *Time,* October 10, 1977, p. 28.

Ogawa, S. Physical fitness and life expectancy of sumo wrestlers. In H. Orimo, K. Shimada, M. Iriki, & D. Maeda (Eds.), *Recent advances in gerontology.* Amsterdam: Excerpta Medica, 1979.

Olson, H.W., Teitelbaum, H., Van Huss, W.D., & Montoye, H.J. Years of sports participation and mortality in college athletes. *Journal of Sports Medicine and Physical Fitness,* 1977, *17,* 321–326.

Ostrow, A.C. Physical activity as it relates to the health of the aged. In N. Datan & N. Lohmann (Eds.), *Transitions of aging.* New York: Academic Press, 1980.

Polednak, A.P. Longevity and cardiovascular mortality among former college athletes. *Circulation,* 1972, *46,* 649–654.

Prout, C. Life expectancy of college oarsmen. *Journal of the American Medical Association,* 1972, *220,* 1709–1711.

Rose, C.L., & Cohen, M.L. Relative importance of physical activity for longevity. *Annals of the New York Academy of Sciences,* 1977, *301,* 671–697.

Rosenthal, R., & Rosnow, R.L. (Eds.). *Artifact in behavioral research.* New York: Academic Press, 1969.

Schaie, K.W. A general model for the study of developmental problems. *Psychological Bulletin,* 1965, *64,* 92–197.

Schmidt, R.A. *Motor control and learning.* Champaign, Ill.: Human Kinetics, 1982.

Shephard, R.J. *Physical activity and aging.* Chicago: Year Book Medical Publishers, 1978.

3

Age-Related Changes in Physical Fitness, Psychomotor Performance, and Personality

Motor development is an emerging academic discipline dedicated to understanding, predicting, and modifying the acquisition and control of movement across the life cycle. Historically, motor development research has focused mainly on a description of those variables thought to govern the large and progressive refinements in motor skill that are most evident prior to adulthood. Only recently has there been a concerted effort by gerontologists, physical educators, psychologists, and others toward understanding motor development across the entire life cycle. Their research efforts have focused primarily on aging effects, and thus, there may be an implicit assumption that their studies are the building blocks of a discipline centered on decline. Unfortunately, research studies directed toward aging effects and human movement seem, for the most part, to bear out this assumption.

A persistent finding in the motor skills literature is the apparent decline during adulthood in almost all motor performance parameters related to participation in physical activity. For example, one of the most ubiquitous changes observed in human performance is the increasing slowness of human behavior with advancing age. This slowness is not limited to simple motor responses commonly reported in the RT literature, but affects complex forms of behavior as well.

In this chapter, I will overview what is known about age-related changes in physical fitness, psychomotor performance, and personality. It will become clear to the reader that, at this point, we lack adequate scientific information regarding the extent to which these changes are inevitable manifestations of biological aging and/or are intertwined with the increasingly sedentary life-styles that people pursue as they grow older.

PHYSICAL FITNESS

A book on psychological perspectives of physical activity and the older adult must still view physical activity holistically: with the

39

understanding that participation in physical activity is dictated by physical conditioning, fitness, and ability as well as appropriate incentives, attitudes, and role expectations. Older adults often approach physical activity with the notion that they are too old to be physically active, and that, in fact, it is "natural" to progressively disengage from physical activity and exercise as one advances in age. These negative attitudes stem, in part, from the common observation that one's level of physical fitness appears to progressively deteriorate with advancing age.

Clarke (1977) has broadly defined physical fitness as:

> [The] ability to carry out daily tasks with vigor and alertness, without undue fatigue, and with ample energy to enjoy leisure-time pursuits and to meet unusual situations and unforeseen circumstances (p. 2).

Within this framework, one can view physical fitness in terms of circulatory-respiratory efficiency, muscular strength and muscular endurance, flexibility, and neuromuscular integrity. These components are not static or predetermined. Rather, the right genes, adequate training, proper diet and sleep, and the right mental attitude all favorably impact on the fitness status of the human organism.

It can be argued that the fitness status of older Americans is a major determinant of their initial propensity toward physical activity participation. Furthermore, one needs to develop a concomitant level of fitness to sustain participation in physical activity and to achieve success. Thus, our level of physical fitness may ultimately interact with the mental health benefits we derive from physical activity participation.

Cardiorespiratory Efficiency

Although there is not total agreement, physical fitness has most often been defined in terms of the maximum level of physical work that the individual is capable of performing. Physical work capacity is a measure of aerobic capacity, and is usually translated as milliliters of oxygen consumption per kilogram of body weight per minute while performing in the laboratory on a treadmill or bicycle ergometer.

It is generally reported that there is a 10 percent decline in maximum oxygen intake ($\dot{V}O_{2\,max}$) per decade of life after the midtwenties among sedentary individuals (Astrand & Rodahl, 1977; Shephard & Sidney, 1979). An overview of 17 cross-sectional studies and 700 observations by Dehn and Bruce (1972) and an overview of cross-sectional research on men aged 20-60 by Hodgson and Buskirk (1977) suggest an annual average decline in $\dot{V}O_{2max}$ of 0.40-0.45 ml/kg/min. Decrements in $\dot{V}O_{2max}$ among sedentary women appear to be slighly less than values reported for sedentary men across chronological age (Espenschade & Eckert, 1980; Hodgson & Buskirk, 1977), leading to a progressively diminished work differential between the sexes.

Longitudinal data on women presented by Voight, Bruce, Kusumi, Pettet, Nilson, Whitkanack, and Tapia (1975) and by Plowman, Drinkwater, and Horvath (1979), as well as longitudinal data overviewed by Hodgson and Buskirk (1977), suggest that the rate of decline in $\dot{V}O_{2max}$ is greater and less uniform than one is led to believe by cross-sectional research. Figure 3-1 contrasts longitudinal $\dot{V}O_{2max}$ data obtained by Plowman and co-workers for five age groups retested after 6 years, with their original cross-sectional $\dot{V}O_{2max}$ data (Drinkwater, Horvath, & Wells, 1975) obtained for these same subjects. Although Dehn and Bruce (1972) indicated that cross-sectional studies are likely to attract cohorts who are physically more fit (and thus distort $\dot{V}O_{2max}$ declines in relation to age), the data from Plowman and co-workers do not reveal differences in $\dot{V}O_{2max}$ decline among female subjects initially categorized as occupationally active or sedentary. Furthermore, Voight and co-workers (1975) noted that the 50 percent subject attrition in their 3.6-year longitudinal study was due, in large part, to the unavailability for retesting of many disease-impaired individuals.

Some exercise scientists have not endorsed $\dot{V}O_{2max}$ as the most valid measure of physical fitness. It appears to have a high genetic component (Astrand, 1968; Spirduso, in press), a conclusion endorsed by Klissouras,

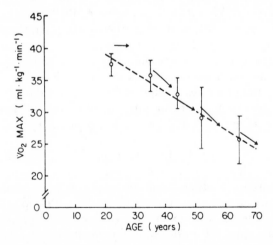

Figure 3-1. Longitudinal (→) changes in $\dot{V}O_{2\,max}$ for five age groups in relation to the means (O), 95% confidence intervals, and regression line (---) for cross-sectional data derived from the original Drinkwater, Horvath, and Wells (1975) study. (From Plowman, S.A., Drinkwater, B.L., & Horvath, S.M. Age and aerobic power in women: A longitudinal study. *Journal of Gerontology*, 1979, *34*, 514. Copyright © 1979 by the Gerontological Society of America. Reprinted by permission.)

41

Pirnay, and Petit (1973) in their cross-sectional $\dot{V}O_{2max}$ data on monozygotic and dizygotic twins aged 9–52. Thus, $\dot{V}O_{2max}$ may not be a sensitive indicator of training, and training, in most cases, does not appear to increase $\dot{V}O_{2max}$ more than 10–20 percent (Astrand, 1968).

There is also considerable controversy regarding the factors that limit maximal performance among old people. Fear of overexertion, muscular weakness, electrocardiographic (ECG) abnormalities, and poor motivation may all interact with observed age-related declines in oxygen transport (Shephard & Sidney, 1979). An investigator is often reluctant to push an elderly subject to exhaustion, particularly since an old person is brought closer to a maximum effort than a young person for a given work load (Shephard & Sidney, 1979). Thus, $\dot{V}O_{2max}$ values in the elderly are frequently estimated using submaximal tests such as the bench step and 12-minute run; however, results derived from submaximal tests on physical work capacity and aging have been contradictory (Bassey, 1978).

Besides $\dot{V}O_{2max}$, there have been other cardiorespiratory changes reported related to aging. Although resting heart rate shows little alteration with advancing age, the maximal heart rate decreases regularly throughout the adult years (Clarke, 1977; deVries, 1977; Drinkwater et al., 1975). Figure 3-2 contasts longitudinal maximal heart rate data obtained by Plowman and co-workers (1979) for five age groups retested after 6 years, with their original cross-sectional maximal heart rate data (Drinkwater et al., 1975) obtained for these same individuals.

Blood volume and total hemoglobin appear to be independent of age, both at rest and under maximal work (Shephard & Sidney, 1979). The maximum output of the heart is diminished among old people (deVries, 1977; Smith, 1981), and their concentration of lactic acid after maximal exertion appears less than that for young people (Shephard & Sidney, 1979).

Respiratory efficiency declines with age. This is evident by the decreased elasticity of the thoracic cage and chest wall, weakened intercostal muscles, inefficient emptying of the lungs, and increased rigidity of internal lung structures (Clarke, 1977; Piscopo, 1981).

For an excellent, more extensive overview of cardiorespiratory function and aging, the reader should consult *Physical Activity and Aging* (Shephard, 1978).

Muscular Strength and Endurance

Muscular strength refers to the strength of the muscles evident in a single maximum contraction. Muscular endurance is defined as the capacity of the muscles to perform continuous work (Clarke, 1977). Both muscular strength and muscular endurance are important components of physical fitness. Compared to other measures of physical fitness,

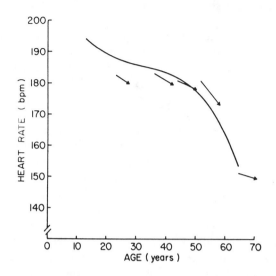

Figure 3-2. Longitudinal (→) changes in maximal heart rate for five age groups in relation to the best-fitting curve for the original cross-sectional data on maximal heart rate vs. age reported by Drinkwater, Horvath, and Wells (1975). (From Plowman, S.A., Drinkwater, B.L., & Horvath, S.M. Age and aerobic power in women: A longitudinal study. *Journal of Gerontology*, 1979, *34*, 515. Copyright © 1979 by the Gerontological Society of America. Reprinted by permission.)

muscular strength seems to be retained for longer periods of time with aging (Hodgson & Buskirk, 1977; Serfass, 1980).

In an early study, Burke, Tuttle, Thompson, Janney, and Weber (1953) examined the grip strength and grip strength endurance (using a hand dynamometer) of 311 males ranging in age from 12 to 79 years. Their data indicated a rapid increase in both strength variables from 12 to 25 years, followed by a gradual decline across age which became more pronounced after 70 years. Similar findings were noted for 218 males, aged 20–89, who were tested for static strength as part of the Baltimore Longitudinal Study (Shock & Norris, 1970). Data on 83 healthy females, aged 19–65, also indicated a significant linear decrease in static grip strength as a function of chronological age (Petrofsky, Burse, & Lind, 1975). In addition, Montoye and Lamphiear (1977) presented data on grip strength (dynamometer) and arm strength (cable pull) for 3,163 males and 3,345 females, aged 10–69, as part of their long-term study of an entire community. Their results suggested little decline in grip strength or arm strength from 20 to 50 years, with more pronounced decrements evident after the age of 50. The authors cautioned that age-related changes in body size and weight should be partialed out from age-based strength data.

Thus, it would seem that the most significant declines in grip strength and endurance occur during the older adult years. Harris (1977) and Astrand and Rodahl (1977) noted that the greatest loss in muscular strength with advancing age occurs in the leg and trunk muscles. Available physiological evidence, however, points to the dedifferentiation of muscle with aging (Fitts, 1981).

It has been proposed (e.g., McCarter, 1978) that adult skeletal muscle is composed of at least three distinct fiber types: type I (slow-twitch, high-oxidative fiber), type IIA (fast-twitch, high-oxidative fiber), and type IIB (fast-twitch, low-oxidative fiber). While the IIB/IIA fiber ratio remains unaltered with increasing age, there is a greater age-related loss in the fast type II fiber relative to type I fiber (Fitts, 1981). Fast-twitch muscles are used for quick, all-out contractions, while slow-twitch fibers are called into play during prolonged, continuous muscular activity (Piscopo, 1981). Thus, the greater age decline in fast-twitch fibers may partially account for observed age-related declines in motor RT, while the less evident decline in type I fiber may be correlated with the more gradual age-related declines observed for muscular endurance. These observations are, of course, based on the assumption that we can readily define three discrete muscle fiber types. It may be more logical to posit a continuum of fiber types in which differentiation is not so readily apparent.

Cross-sectional data on age differences in muscular strength and endurance may underestimate age effects. Previous physical activity involvement, health status, variations in body dimensions, and other factors need to be carefully controlled if aging effects are to be interpretable.

Flexibility

Flexibility, or adequate range of joint motion, is an essential ingredient in the physical fitness of older people. For many years, flexibility was viewed as a therapeutic measure. Today, there is greater recognition of the importance of adequate flexibility in the overall fitness status of the individual.

Although there is a paucity of research on aging and flexibility, the available literature suggests a gradual loss in range of joint motion (Adrian, 1981; Serfass, 1980). Decreased flexibility with age is probably the result of combined histological and morphological changes in the components of the joint, including cartilage, ligaments, and tendons. The greater calcification of cartilage and surrounding tissue, the shortening of muscles, increased tension and anxiety, and the prevalence of arthritic and other orthopedic conditions all contribute to reduced flexibility (Piscopo, 1981). However, as Adrian (1981) has stated, "there is no evidence that biological aging processes cause this decrease in flexibility, since most research links degenerative diseases with loss of flexibility" (p. 55).

Activities of daily life, sports, and other forms of recreational activities all require adequate range of joint motion. Although age-related declines in flexibility seem to be joint specific, the greatest declines appear to be noted in movements not habitually performed by older people (Adrian, 1981). Thus, although the aging joint causes instability and some loss of mobility (Shephard & Sidney, 1979), these effects may not prevent older persons from functionally completing daily routines (Adrian, 1981). Nevertheless, the loss of joint motion may reduce the older person's potential to excel and may increase his/her proneness toward injury while performing in sport and related physical activities (Humphrey, 1981).

Discussion

The evidence suggests age-related declines in cardiorespiratory efficiency, muscular strength and endurance, and joint range of motion—all essential elements of physical fitness. It is not clear, however, to what extent these changes are a function of age, disease, or disuse and inactivity. For example, 3 weeks of bed rest will bring about some of these changes in well-conditioned young subjects (deVries, 1977). Cardiovascular deconditioning studies during chair rest (Lamb, Johnson, & Stevens, 1964) and bed rest (see Serfass, 1980, for an overview) and the deteriorating effects of weightlessness and inactivity during space flight confirm the notion that declines in physical fitness are related to factors other than age. In addition, as I shall discuss in Chapter 4, many of the age-related declines in physical fitness can be deterred through training. Thus, we need to be extremely cautious when interpreting age differences in physical fitness as aging effects.

Many textbooks written on motor behavior and on psychology and physical activity fail to address the important relationship of physical fitness to motor performance. Advancing age and the increased probability of disease make it extremely difficult for many older people to renew their commitment toward being physically active. The burden is then placed on the trained professional to isolate the effects of inactivity and disinterest from pathology if he/she is to successfully develop and promote programs of physical activity for older people.

PSYCHOMOTOR PERFORMANCE

With advancing age, psychomotor performance becomes slower and more inconsistent. Both interindividual and intraindividual performance variability increase with age.

For example, field-based data (see Table 3-1) obtained on men's records for Masters running speeds in track events, compiled by Mundle (1979) and analyzed by Stones and Kozma (1980), suggest a decline in running speed with advancing age. Stones and Kozma, using an exponential model to fit performance time to age, found that the rate of age decline in running performance was greater for middle- and longer-distance events than for sprints and that, generally, performance variability increased with advancing age.

Table 3-1

Median Record Performances (in seconds) Associated with Various Age Intervals and Event Distances[a]

Event distance	Age interval (years)						
	40–44	45–49	50–54	55–59	60–64	65–69	70–74
100 yards	9.8 (0.19)	10.5 (0.22)	10.6 (0.18)	10.7 (0.05)	12.1 (0.58)	12.3 (0.11)	13.7 (0.05)
100 m	11.0 (0.16)	11.3 (0.12)	11.6 (0.36)	11.6 (0.12)	12.4 (0.46)	13.5 (0.27)	14.6 (0.35)
200 m	22.7 (0.45)	23.2 (0.47)	23.6 (0.14)	24.7 (1.63)	25.5 (0.86)	28.3 (0.45)	30.2 (0.79)
400 m	50.5 (1.15)	52.1 (0.26)	53.9 (0.70)	56.8 (2.83)	59.7 (1.27)	65.8 (3.08)	68.1 (1.70)
800 m	116.3 (1.97)	118.4 (0.89)	124.0 (4.82)	134.5 (2.65)	142.8 (3.68)	150.2 (4.63)	155.8 (1.13)
1,500 m	238.8 (3.54)	250.4 (4.15)	255.0 (4.59)	268.0 (3.64)	291.3 (4.72)	309.4 (10.45)	326.1 (4.00)
1 mile	261.5 (3.66)	272.8 (3.05)	289.8 (14.38)	308.5 (14.23)	322.1 (7.11)	341.4 (13.98)	352.3 (19.75)
3,000 m	503.6 (11.65)	529.4 (9.19)	573.7 (11.10)	619.8 (45.14)	641.0 (18.89)	672.8 (42.51)	725.9 (16.07)
5,000 m	860.4 (22.98)	907.4 (24.56)	963.6 (15.83)	989.0 (35.83)	1,058.0 (31.86)	1,143.6 (41.39)	1,205.4 (41.27)
10,000 m	1,751.4 (49.15)	1,893.8 (47.44)	1,956.2 (52.19)	2,024.2 (118.31)	2,176.0 (56.58)	2,356.0 (120.49)	2,656.2 (129.34)
Marathon	8,167.0 (170.57)	8,526.0 (169.01)	8,960.0 (219.58)	9,499.0 (677.57)	10,254.0 (192.37)	10,605.0 (348.25)	11,687.0 (1,482.10)

Note. From "Adult Age Trends in Record Running Performances" by M.J. Stones and A. Kozma, *Experimental Aging Research,* 1980, *6,* 410–411, as adapted from "Masters Records: Men's Records," by P. Mundle, *Runner's World,* 1979, *14.*88-93. Copyright © 1980 by Beach Hill Enterprises, Inc. Reprinted by permission.

[a]Numbers in parentheses indicate standard deviations.

In contrast, Moore (1975) analyzed men's and women's age-group track and field records. Using an exponential model to plot speed against age (see Figure 3-3), Moore found a gradual deterioration in running speed after age 30 across all running distance events, an increase in the age of maximum performance with the distance of the event, a slower rate of deterioration in running speed (by age) at longer distances, and, beyond age 30, a faster rate of deterioration in speed for women than men. Decreased performance (speed) and increased variability as a function of age were also reported by Rahe and Arthur (1975) for men's swimming events.

The Reaction Time–Movement Time Paradigm

In the laboratory, researchers generally fractionate human speed of response (or total response time) into two components: reaction time and movement time. In a typical experiment the subject is asked (1) to release a telegraph key held by the hand when an unanticipated stimulus is presented and (2) to move this hand as rapidly as possible to some target. In this paradigm, RT is typically defined as the measure of time from the presentation of the sudden, unanticipated stimulus to the initiation of the movement. MT is usually defined as the measure of time from the initiation of the response to the completion of the movement. Therefore, total response time is the summation of RT and MT.

The slowness of simple RT with age is "one of the most replicated findings of behavioral change with age" (Birren, Woods, & Williams, 1980, p. 294). In an overview of 26 studies on simple RT and age, Birren and co-workers reported that, on the average, there was a 20 percent difference in RT between 20-year-olds and 60-year-olds.

Using EMG recordings, researchers have suggested that RT can be partitioned into central and peripheral components. Figure 3-4 presents a stylized EMG recording of the critical events that appear to be involved in a simple (single stimulus–single response) RT paradigm. The time from the presentation of the stimulus to the activation of the muscle (i.e., when an evoked potential is recorded from the motor cortex) is typically termed *premotor RT* (Schmidt, 1982; Spirduso, 1980). Within a 200-msec total response time interval, for example, in which a subject (in response to a visual stimulus) quickly releases a microswitch and then depresses another microswitch (MT) in approximately 20 msec, we might expect premotor RT in the agonist or prime mover to approximate 160 msec (Spirduso, 1980). Thus, premotor RT (or the time when the EMG recording is silent) represents a substantial portion of the total response time interval.

In this paradigm, it takes approximately 40 msec for the visual stimulus to evoke a response in the occipital cortex. Most of the remaining 120 msec of premotor RT is thought to represent central

47

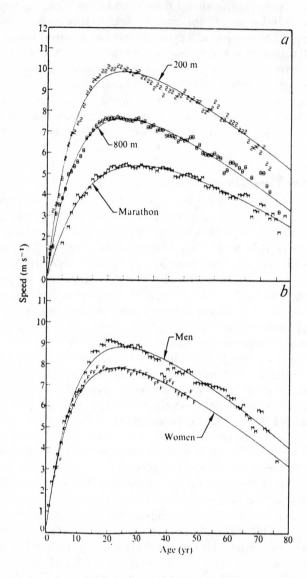

Figure 3-3. Exponential curves for (a) men's age-group track records in 200 m, 800 m, and the marathon, and (b) age-group track records for men and women in 400 m. (From Moore, D.H. A study of age group track and field records to relate age and running speed. *Nature*, 1975, *253*, 264, as adapted from data compiled by Shepard, J., Donavan, W., & Mundle, P. Age records 1974. *Track and Field News Press*, Los Altos, Calif., 1974, and by Reel, V. *Women's Track and Field World*. Claremont, Calif. Copyright © 1975 by Macmillan Journals Limited. Reprinted by permission.)

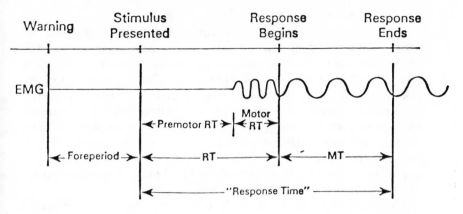

Figure 3-4. Stylized EMG record of muscle depicting the critical events involved in RT paradigm. (From Schmidt, R.A. *Motor control and learning.* Champaign, Ill.: Human Kinetics, 1982. Copyright © 1982 by Richard A. Schmidt. Reprinted by permission.)

information-processing time in which the integrity of the central nervous system is invoked (Spirduso, 1980). There seems to be a general consensus that this central component is predominantly responsible for observed age-related decrements in RT. However, most of the earlier reported data on RT and aging do not lend themselves to a component analysis of RT.

As can be seen in Figure 3-4, the time interval from the first recorded EMG activity to finger movement is termed *motor RT* (Schmidt, 1982) and includes both nerve conduction time and muscle contractile time (Spirduso, 1980). The time it takes from the initiation of the response (e.g., to release a key or microswitch) to the completion of the response (e.g., to depress another key) is MT. Muscle contractile time plus MT are viewed as peripheral components in this RT paradigm.

Although MT can be controlled to a few milliseconds in the laboratory, most physical activities demand considerably longer MT intervals. Correlation coefficients between MT and RT have generally been found to be low, suggesting that the processes underlying one's ability to react quickly are different from those underlying the ability to move quickly once the reaction is made. MT is often studied in skills research because of its potential applicability to understanding sport and related physical activity movements. On the other hand, while RT has some bearing on physical activity performance, it is frequently studied in the laboratory because it can serve as a controlled measure of cognitive processes (such as decision making and response programming) that underlie skillful performance (Schmidt, 1982).

49

An Information-processing Model

One of the more popular and systematic approaches to studying the sensory-motor system has been to conceptualize human skillful performance in terms of an information-processing model. This model depicts humans as processors of information. The execution of a motor response is thought to involve a series of stages that involve the acceptance, storage, and processing of information before effector mechanisms are actuated. Information seems to follow through these stages, with each stage presumably characterized by higher levels of abstraction (Hoyer & Plude, 1980). These stages can occur serially (i.e., sequentially) or simultaneously (Schmidt, 1982). This information-processing model is illustrated in Figure 3-5.

The simple RT paradigm can be discussed within an information-processing framework. It takes approximately 40 msec for a visual stimulus to be translated by peripheral receptors into electrochemical impulses and to evoke a response in the occipital cortex (*preperceptual processes*) during a 200-msec response time interval. This procedure has been termed detection, because environmental changes are coded into nervous impulses related to the characteristics of the visual stimulus. These impulses are stored briefly in what has been termed a short-term sensory store (STSS) (Stelmach & Diewert, 1977). This peripheral level of processing is thought to be a memory system in which large amounts of information are stored for very brief periods of time. It is not clear if separate STSS systems exist for each sense modality (Schmidt, 1982); there is some evidence (Walsh & Thompson, 1978) that the visual storage capacity of old subjects is not as great as that for young subjects.

Once the environmental stimuli are detected they must be recognized or evaluated (Stelmach & Diewert, 1977); that is, only relevant information in the STSS must be selected for further processing (through selective attention). If one takes the position that perception involves the recognition or evaluation of information, then *perceptual processes* can be viewed as central rather than peripheral (Stelmach & Diewert, 1977): perceptual processes invoke the central nervous system into action.

During the *response-selection stage,* the individual must decide on a course of action. A decision can be made not to respond or to select a response(s) from a large number of alternatives. The choice RT paradigm (i.e., more than one stimulus–more than one response required) has frequently been used to study information processing during this stage. It is well known (Hick's law) that the relationship between choice RT and the logarithm to the base two of the number of stimulus-response alternatives is linear. In other words, there seems to be a linear relationship between the amount of information that must be processed (the logarithm of the number of stimulus-response alternatives) and the time required to make a decision (Schmidt, 1982). Thus, as Schmidt has

50

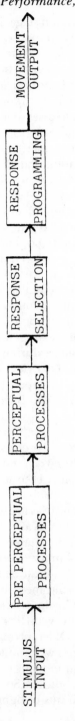

Figure 3-5. An information-processing model of human performance. (Based on Schmidt, 1982, and Stelmach and Diewert, 1977.)

51

observed, during the response-selection stage the individual attempts to reduce uncertainty about alternative responses to a given stimulus. The choice RT paradigm has been used to study the impact of aging on decision time during this response-selection stage.

Once a response has been selected, the individual must organize, plan, and initiate movement. During the *response-programming stage*, information must be translated into a set of muscular actions. Memory (stored information) is brought into play (as it is in the preceding stages of this model), and the duration of the response-programming stage appears to be related to the duration and complexity of the response required (Schmidt, 1982).

The information-processing model described here provides a systematic, behavioral approach to conceptualizing human movement in which inferences are made regarding central nervous system action through "input regulation–output observation" (Marteniuk, 1976). There seems to be some consensus, at least in terms of simple RT, that slowness due to aging lies in the central nervous system and occurs between the time at which sensory nerve conduction is completed and the time it takes to activate peripheral neuromuscular systems (Botwinick, 1978). Thus, an information-processing model provides a logical framework for identifying what stages during human performance are most affected by aging processes. This viewpoint is not new and has found much support, particularly in papers by Welford (1965), Birren (1974), Stelmach and Diewert (1977), and Birren and co-workers (1980).

Preperceptual Processes

Literature suggests that the decreased processing ability of older adults may be attributable, in part, to reduced detectability. The effects of aging on sensory input have most frequently been studied in relation to visual and auditory systems. As Botwinick (1978) has noted, the literature is very clear—older people do not see or hear as acutely as do younger people.

The decline in visual acuity accelerates after approximately 50 years of age, with the loss most likely attributable to modifications in the crystalline lens and the vitreous humor (Corso, 1971; Smith & Sethi, 1975). The proportion of adults with 20/20 vision diminishes by 75 percent between 60 and 80 years, and the reduced elasticity of the lens produces increasing levels of farsightedness among older people (Kalish, 1982). Changes involving the crystalline lens also affect light transmission and refractoriness. Older people need greater levels of illumination, and they cannot see as well in the dark (Botwinick, 1978). The ability of the eye to accommodate (i.e., discriminate) detail diminishes with age (Corso, 1971; Smith & Sethi, 1975), and there is less ability to adjust to changing amounts of light (Kalish, 1982). There is also a greater narrowing of the peripheral visual field with advancing age (Colavita, 1978; Kalish, 1982).

With respect to audition, Botwinick (1978) stated that hearing loss should not be confused with an increase in cautious behavior and a decrease in attentive behavior among old people. Nevertheless, as with vision, there is a loss of auditory acuity with advancing age known as presbycusis. The loss of acuity is more extensive for higher-range tones (Botwinick, 1978; Colavita, 1978; Kalish, 1982), and older people have poorer discrimination among tones (Botwinick, 1978). Hearing impairment appears to be more common than visual impairment after 65 years, and older people have greater difficulty understanding speech (particularly in noisy environments) because of hearing problems (Corso, 1971; Kalish, 1982).

Information is more limited on other sense modalities with aging, particularly those modalities having special relevance to gross motor performance. Reduced eye oscillation time and decreased nausea associated with vertical stimulation of the semicircular canals suggest age declines in vestibular mechanisms (Noble, 1978). These vestibular changes lead to declines in one's sense of body position and in balance. Falls in the elderly are common and are associated with frequent injuries, and sometimes death. Postural sway is more evident in older people and is believed to be due to less control of postural muscles and diminished efficiency of postural reflexes (Hasselkus & Shambes, 1975; Overstall, Exton-Smith, Imms, & Johnson, 1977).

There is some evidence that touch sensitivity (Thompson, Axelrod, & Cohen, 1965) and pain sensitivity (Botwinick, 1978; Corso, 1971; Smith & Sethi, 1975) decline with advancing age. However, pain sensitivity appears to be specific to the body part in question and to the type of stimulus used to elicit a response (Corso, 1971). In addition, the validity of using self-report measures of pain sensitivity among older people may be questionable (Kalish, 1982). Although pain tolerance may be a desirable attribute among exercise participants, it is doubtful that pain sensitivity studies based on dental cavity preparations or on the use of external heat have much bearing on understanding pain tolerance levels among exercisers.

Although there is a general decline in sensory processes with advancing age, the onset and rate of decline of these functions appear to vary both between and within sensory modalities (Corso, 1971). Peripheral changes in various sensory modalities may only account for a small proportion of the deterioration observed in premotor RT, at least in terms of simple RT (Weiss, 1965). Research reviewed by Botwinick (1965, 1978) clearly demonstrated that a slowing of peripheral nerve conduction velocity did not appreciably account for increases in RT with age. When Botwinick (1972) equated loud tone stimuli with the detection abilities of subjects, there was still evidence for the deterioration of RT with age. There is also evidence that some reflexes (e.g., patellar tendon, Achilles tendon) deteriorate very little with age (Spirduso, in press). All of these findings point to the notion that central mechanisms, rather than peripheral mechanisms, are responsible for psychomotor slowing and aging.

Perception and Attention

Perceptual mechanisms, within an information-processing framework, enable the individual to recognize or evaluate information through a process of selective attention—that is through an ability to separate relevant from irrelevant information. Perceptual processing is constrained by both space (the amount of information that can be processed) and time, (temporal differences in the rate of processing) (Hoyer & Plude, 1980).

There are few age differences in recognizing two-dimensional figures unless viewing conditions are hindered by poor illumination, inadequate contrast, or other factors (Noble, 1978). Older subjects, however, have more difficulty perceiving embedded (hidden) figures (Corso, 1971; Markus, 1971). In addition, Rotella and Bunker (1978a) reported that field-independent older tennis players appear to react more quickly than field-dependent older tennis players, although this study may have confounded field independency-dependency with initial tennis skill levels.

Most investigations of age-related changes in perceptual processing have focused on time constraints rather than spatial constraints. For example, in studies of masking (rapid sequential presentation of two visual stimuli leading to the occlusion of one of the stimuli), there is a general tendency for older age groups to require longer critical periods to escape masking effects (Birren et al., 1980; Hoyer & Plude, 1980). In addition, in studies of critical flicker fusion (in which the viewer is presented a sequence of rapidly flashing lights), it takes a higher rate of on-off flickering for younger subjects to perceive a steady stream of light than for older subjects (Botwinick, 1978; Corso, 1971). It has been suggested that the first light stimulus may persist longer in the central nervous system of older people, particularly when interstimulus sequences are very short (Botwinick, 1978).

Stelmach and Diewert (1977) indicated that recognition of information may decline with age, in part, because of the poorer attentional abilities evident with advancing age. Attentional ability might be defined as a limited, selective capacity (or resource) to address particular stimuli or information. From an information-processing perspective, one's ability to attend is affected by a limited central-processing capacity that is particularly evident when two similar tasks (in terms of receptor-effector systems) are performed simultaneously (Etzel, 1979; Marteniuk, 1976; Schmidt, 1982). Although attention demands appear to be made during all stages of processing, Schmidt (1982) has suggested that attentional demands become progressively greater as processing comes closer to a response, at least in terms of RT. In a review of literature, Hoyer and Plude (1980) concluded that older people may have more difficulty ignoring irrelevant information and that there are age-related declines in the capacity of attention.

It has been hypothesized that an optimal level of central nervous system activity underlies maximal performance, and that increasing autonomic activity (arousal), to an extent, promotes optimal central nervous system activity (Marteniuk, 1976). The inverted-U hypothesis, originally based on the work of Yerkes and Dodson (1908) on mice, has been extended to suggest that a curvilinear relationship (inverted U) exists between arousal and gross motor performance. Although this relationship remains to be adequately tested in the realm of physical activity, the hypothesis does suggest that there may be an optimal level of arousal specific to each motor task, and that excessive arousal (or what I prefer to call excessive state anxiety*) leads to a decrement in performance. This decline in performance has been linked to possible alterations in the attentional capacities of the subject. Task complexity, uncertainty, meaningfulness, and variation may all mediate state anxiety, but the important point appears to be that elevated levels of anxiety (based on perceived stress) may lead to greater distractibility, an excessive narrowing of attentional focus, and a redirection of attention toward task-irrelevant cues (Landers, 1980; Nideffer, 1981). If this is all true, then perhaps age differences in performance observed on RT tasks may be due, in part, to higher levels of state anxiety present among older subjects during performance.

Welford (1965, 1969) originally proposed that, under high arousal, there was increased "noise" in the central nervous system due to the increased spontaneous but random firing of cortical cells. This elevation in neural activity produced interference, and fewer cells were left to carry appropriate information. Welford (1965) further noted that common, everyday observations would suggest that many older people are tense and anxious and thus, perhaps, less attentive.

Unfortunately, traditional autonomic measures of arousal (e.g., heart rate, galvanic skin response) do not correlate well with self-report measures of state anxiety, leading investigators to view state anxiety as multidimensional (e.g., Endler, 1977). More creative approaches are needed to identify the impact of anxiety on age-related differences in

---

*State anxiety refers to transitory levels of nervousness or worry that may be temporary or chronically based. State anxiety has at least two modes of expression: a cognitive mode and a somatic mode. Excessive arousal may or may not be symptomatic of high levels of state anxiety.

attention. For example, Weinberg and Hunt's (1976) isolation of state anxiety performance effects through EMG analysis, coupled with Pfefferbaum, Ford, Roth, Hopkins, and Kopell's (1979) analysis of attention based on event-related brain potential (ERP) data, would seem to offer some interesting solutions to understanding the effects of anxiety on age-related changes in attention.

Schmidt (1982) speculated that high levels of arousal might hinder motor performance on tasks that required fine control, steadiness, and/or rapid decisions based on a number of alternatives. A cursory observation of motor tasks selected to study aging effects suggests that they often meet one or more of these criteria. Tests of power that are self-paced and have no time limits (and that, perhaps, are less affected by arousal conditions) show less marked age declines (Noble, 1978). We must be careful not to overestimate age-related declines in human motor performance based on the limited types of motor tasks that have been employed.

There have been other strategies used to understand why older people have more difficulty performing motor tasks requiring high levels of attention. Efforts to link electroencephalographic (EEG) brain wave activity to the question of increased slowing with age have not been very successful (e.g., Botwinick & Thompson, 1968; Woodruff & Kramer, 1979). Also, signal detection theory has been applied to studies of aging (e.g., Craik, 1969), in which subjects are asked to detect or discriminate noise plus a signal from just noise. It has been found that stressful conditions lead to more false alarms, impair the detection of information, and may lead to errors of commission rather than omission (Marteniuk, 1976). Thus, there may be a relationship between arousal and signal detection theory in that, as Welford (1965) has suggested, under aroused conditions a signal must be detected from "noisy" central nervous system activity. However, confidence, cautiousness, motivational state, vigilance, and other characteristics of the subject also need to be carefully controlled in this line of research. As Schmidt (1982) has observed, signal detection theory has not been applied very much to motor behavior research.

Botwinick (1978) proposed that the preparatory interval, or foreperiod, (the time from when a warning signal is presented to the onset of the stimulus) in a RT–MT paradigm differentially affects premotor RT based on age. However, although Loveless and Sanford (1974) found that older people were especially slow at the longest foreperiods selected, they felt that this was due to an inability to initiate rather than to maintain preparation, a contention supported by the findings of Gottsdanker (1980).

Response Selection

Once information has been evaluated (based on perceptual mechanisms), the individual must decide on a course of action. The decision may be not to respond or to select a response(s) from a large number of alternatives. Decision processes have frequently been examined in the laboratory via the choice RT paradigm, in which the potential exists for establishing multiple stimuli–multiple response patterns under controlled conditions. One of the most important findings resulting from this line of research is Hick's law, which suggests a linear relationship between the amount of information that must be processed to make a decision (i.e., the logarithm of the number of stimulus-response alternatives) and the time required to make that decision (Schmidt, 1982). When the number of stimulus-response alternatives is doubled, choice RT appears to increase by a constant amount. However, this relationship is affected by the degree of stimulus-response compatibility and the amount of practice allowed on the task (Schmidt, 1982), and also may be affected by the ages of the subjects under investigation.

One of the most persistent findings in the research literature is that differences in RT between young and old become more magnified with increasingly more complex choice RT tasks. Illustrative of this phenomenon are data (see Figure 3-6) by Stern, Oster, and Newport (1980) who found that task demand accounted for 40 percent of the variance in decision (reaction) time among male and female adults (ranging in average age from 20 to 75 years). However, the task-demand effect for decision time was mostly attributable to the difference in response between the reverse-choice task (a task in which a left light signaled a right-finger response and the right light a left-finger response) and all other tasks. These findings are consistent with a review by Cerella, Poon, and Williams (1980), who found that data from 18 studies encompassing a wide variety of information-processing tasks supported the hypothesis that more complex tasks result in greater performance deficits for the elderly.

Increasingly more complex choice RT tasks seem to contain larger cognitive requirements. Attempts to describe an aging effect have, for example, considered the possibility that there are age-related declines in the memory access required for performing more complex tasks (Cerella et al., 1980; Marteniuk, 1974). Botwinick (1978) suggested that the long stimuli exposure durations in complex tasks may promote disproportionate slowing among the elderly because of the increased cautiousness with which they approach these tasks. Stelmach and Diewert (1977) speculated that increased choice RT with age might simply be a function of increased simple RT with age. However, there appears to be a general consensus (e.g., Cerella et al., 1980) that the slower

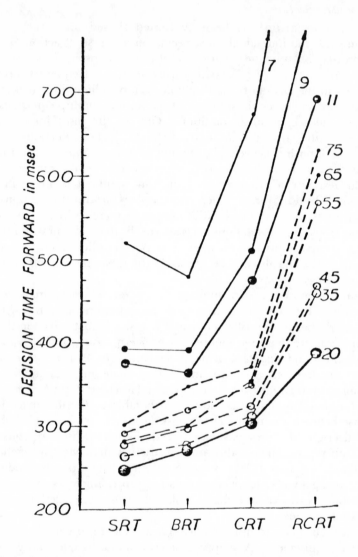

Figure 3-6. Decision time forward as a function of age. (Numbers next to lines on graph refer to average age of men and women in each group. SRT = simple reaction time; BRT = bilateral reaction time; CRT = choice reaction time; RCRT = reverse choice reaction time. From Stern, J.A., Oster, P.J., & Newport, K. Reaction time measures, hemispheric specialization, and age. In L.W. Poon (Ed.), *Aging in the 1980s*. Washington, D.C.: American Psychological Association, 1980. Copyright © 1980 by the American Psychological Association. Reprinted by permission of the publisher and author.)

RT of older subjects on increasingly more complex tasks represents a decline in central processes, although the mechanisms involved await further investigation. It may be that these mechanisms lie in the response-programming stage.

Response Programming

During the response-programming stage, information must be translated into a set of muscular actions. However, as Stelmach and Diewert (1977) noted, there has been little systematic research toward determining a person's ability to organize or plan movement, especially with regard to age changes.

Experimenters have consistently shown that the RT to the second of two almost simultaneously occurring stimuli is almost always greater than the RT to the first stimulus in the absence of the second stimulus (Marteniuk, 1976; Schmidt, 1982). This phenomenon has been termed the *psychological refractory period*. The cause of this delay appears to lie in central rather than peripheral mechanisms. A single-channel hypothesis, originally proposed by Welford (1952), suggested that the decision mechanism was a single channel in which only a single signal could be processed at one time. Although the single-channel hypothesis is currently viewed as too simplistic in explaining complex motor behavior (Marteniuk, 1976), the existence of psychological refractoriness has not been refuted. In fact, this phenomenon is even more apparent in elderly subjects (Botwinick, 1978, Welford, 1977b). Welford proposed that older people may have more difficulty discriminating repeated signals and/or they may monitor their responses more than young people.

Memory

A dynamic perspective on information processing during movement assumes that information is retained (or stored) for future use during the various stages of processing. The framework or systems involved in this storage have been labeled memory (Schmidt, 1982). It is generally accepted that there are at least three separate memory systems: STSS (discussed earlier in this chapter), short-term memory (STM), and long-term memory (LTM). These three systems differ in terms of the amount and type of information that is stored and the rate of loss of information (Marteniuk, 1976; Schmidt, 1982; Stelmach & Diewert, 1977).

The STSS briefly stores impulses (information) used during detection (preperceptual processes). Although there is evidence that the STSS deteriorates with aging (e.g., Birren et al., 1980; Botwinick, 1978), this decline may have minimal impact on psychomotor slowing; the STSS is the most peripheral level of processing in the information-processing model.

There is evidence that STM efficiency declines with age (Birren et al., 1980; Stelmach & Diewert, 1977). The STM system is thought to be a limited storage capacity system focusing on more abstract information than the STSS (Schmidt, 1982). Although there appears to be only a minimal reduction in STM capacity with advancing age (Birren et al., 1980; Botwinick, 1978), the scan (or item-by-item sequential review) of STM seems to decline with age. Declines in STM efficiency may be due to system interference or an inability to shift attention between incoming information and storage utilization (Stelmach & Diewert, 1977).

The LTM system stores very abstract and complex information gained through practice, and seems to have an almost unlimited capacity to store information for very long periods of time (Schmidt, 1982). As such, the LTM provides us with a capacity to retain motor skills once well learned (e.g., swimming, riding a bicycle). Reviews of research literature by Botwinick (1978) and by Stelmach and Diewert (1977) suggest that age-related declines in LTM (at least in terms of new learning) center more on declines in recall (i.e., the searching and retrieval of stored information) than on declines in recognition (i.e., the matching of stored information without retrieval). However, there may be little decline with age in the retrieval of very old, basic information. The LTM of older people appears to be more susceptible to interference, and older people may have more difficulty consolidating information in the LTM system (Botwinick, 1978; Stelmach & Diewert, 1977).

Discussion

An information-processing model of human movement is but a first step in the systematic effort to uncover the mechanisms by which psychomotor speed declines with age. Models serve important purposes. A good model provides a clear outline or graphic framework for the systematic investigation of testable hypotheses and theories. As such, the information-processing model has been a useful and popular approach toward understanding aging and psychomotor slowing. However, as with any model, there are potential drawbacks. A failure to understand these drawbacks could seriously curtail our efforts toward understanding, predicting, and modifying the impact of age on psychomotor performance.

The bulk of research directed toward the question of psychomotor slowing with age has focused on the RT–MT paradigm. The study of RT in highly controlled, laboratory settings has led us to a consensus (to date) that the mechanisms responsible for age-related declines in RT lie in the central nervous system. Thus, RT-directed research has been useful in suggesting that cognitive (mental) processes underly the decline in psychomotor slowing with advancing age. However, the nature or specifications of these cognitive processes need to be identified through theory development and testing.

More than 10 years ago, the noted gerontologist James Birren (1970) outlined a number of theories that had been proposed to account, in part, for psychomotor slowing with age. These, and other theoretical explanations mentioned in this chapter, are presented in Figure 3-7. Some (or perhaps all) of these theories focus on neurophysiological changes with age. Other theories seem to focus on age-related changes in "surface" personality characteristics such as state anxiety or cautiousness. The important point would seem to be, however, that only by the systematic testing of these theories through the development of creative research designs can we ultimately hope to make predictive statements about the impact of aging on RT.

We should not lose sight of the fact that RT is but a peripheral component to understanding many complex motor skills inherent in physical activity. Thus, while an information-processing model has been useful in conceptualizing the impact of age on RT in controlled, laboratory settings, motor behavior researchers (e.g., Schmidt, 1982) tell us that an information-processing perspective falls far short of explaining the detection of error and execution of corrective actions during rapid movement. I find it surprising, for example, that little, if any, research has been directed toward understanding age-related changes in generalized motor programs, or "engram" formations (Ager, White, Mayberry, Crist, & Conrad, 1981), thought to underly the control of complex movement.

A well-known phenomenon that occurs during motor performance is the so-called speed-accuracy trade-off (e.g., Marteniuk, 1976; Schmidt, 1982). It is surprising that those (few) studies that have focused on movement time and aging have not controlled for the potential confounding affects of accuracy when examining the impact of age on psychomotor speed. It has been documented (see Welford, 1977a, for a review) that the elderly are often more cautious (particularly in a laboratory environment) and more unwilling to make errors in skilled performance than younger subjects. Thus, they sometimes adopt alternative strategies when asked to execute movements that are couched in terms of trying to be more accurate. To correctly interpret research on psychomotor slowing and aging, accuracy may need to be held constant through experimental manipulation (Schmidt, 1982).

Psychomotor slowing with advancing age appears to be universal to humans. Thus, there is the temptation (e.g., Birren et al., 1980) to try to detect a common set of mechanisms that account for the diffuseness of this phenomenon. However, it is known (e.g., Noble, 1978; Salthouse, 1976) that not all motor activities requiring speeded performance

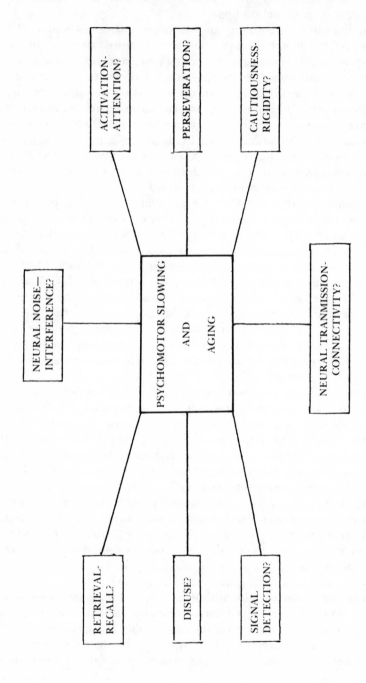

Figure 3-7. Psychomotor slowing and aging: An overview of theoretical directions.

evidence a decline with age at the same rate. The steepest age-related declines may be for paced speed tests having strict time limits. Performance on self-paced tests of power (having no time limits) may show less decline with age (Noble, 1978). In addition, performance on simple RT tasks show only a gradual decline with age (Salthouse, 1976). The fact that individual differences in psychomotor speed become much more prominent with advancing age, and that some age-related declines in psychomotor performance may be retarded through exercise and practice, cannot be overlooked. As Welford (1965) has observed, "human age changes take place in a complex dynamic system in which there are many different detailed mechanisms, only one of which may limit performance in any particular task" (pp. 16-17). Thus, our search for a global theory to explain psychomotor slowing and aging may be the wrong path to follow.

PERSONALITY

The study of human personality has had a history steeped in controversy. This can be attributed, in part, to the complex nature of personality and to the difficulty of studying human personality at a molar or surface level. How we proceed to investigate aging, human personality change, and psychomotor performance must be based on the theoretical orientation(s) that we espouse. We may be naive in using projective techniques, for example, to study personality, if we do not believe that human personality functioning stems, in part, from unconscious, deep-seated, and covert levels of motivation. It will become apparent shortly that the majority of literature on aging, personality change, and psychomotor performance centers around a personality trait approach.

Personality theory is often heavily based on the use of psychological *constructs*, or hypothetical variables (such as "aggression") that have been created to describe an observed behavioral phenomenon. These constructs are usually operationalized, or defined more narrowly, for the purpose of empirical investigation. For example, one might define and study aggression based on the number of electric shocks a subject willingly administers to a confederate in a controlled, laboratory setting. It is apparent, however, that this procedure (i.e., the operationalization of constructs) may limit the potential external validity of human personality investigation.

I have suggested that personality changes with age, such as increased cautiousness or rigidity, may account, in part, for the observed age-related declines in psychomotor speed and performance. Older people bring to any movement activity a history rich in life experiences. As such, it is important to reiterate that older people are more heterogeneous than similar. We must be careful not to stereotype older people as, for example, rigid, cautious, mellow, or cantankerous. Furthermore, bearing in mind that the majority of research studies on personality and aging are based on the use of the cross-sectional research design, we must be careful not to see observed age (or cohort) differences as necessarily indicative of an aging effect on human personality.

Achievement Motivation

Competitive sport and other related physical activities provide an excellent arena for the investigation of achievement-oriented behaviors. Achievement-oriented performances are typically characterized by a standard of excellence whereby success or failure are inevitable outcomes; an element of challenge, generated to some extent by outcome uncertainty; and a willingness of the individual to accept responsibility for the performance outcome (Maehr, 1974). As such, achievement motivation is instrumental to successful performance in physical activity. There has been some suggestion, however, that old people have lower needs for achievement (Botwinick, 1978; Schulz, 1982) and may be less interested in competing.

The study of achievement motivation has had a long and intensive history stemming from McClelland and co-workers' (1953) original work on the need for achievement. Over the last 30 years, research efforts have progressed from an initial effort to validate a modified Thematic Apperception Test, a projective assessment of need achievement, to experimental studies of factors influencing the expression of achievement motivation, to macroanalyses of the role of achievement in economic and social growth, and, finally, to planned programs of intervention leading toward the modification of achievement motivation.

Atkinson's (e.g., Atkinson, 1958; Atkinson & Feather, 1966) research on achievement motivation ultimately led to the theory that achievement-oriented performances arouse within the individual two conflicting response tendencies: the tendency to achieve success and the tendency to avoid failure. These response tendencies are presumed to be multiplicative functions of the individual's relatively stable predispositions (or motives) toward achieving success or avoiding failure, the individual's real and perceived expectancies of experiencing success/failure, and the incentive value(s) the individual placed on achieving success or avoiding failure. While this theory has been difficult to apply and verify in sport and physical activity, it nevertheless gave recognition to the complex interactions between the person and his/her perceived environment that are fundamental to achievement expression.

Developmental examinations of achievement motivation in relation to physical activity have been limited primarily to those factors influencing the socialization of achievement expression in children (e.g., Veroff, 1969). There has been no systematic effort toward developing a life-span perspective on achievement motivation (Maehr & Kleiber, 1980). Given that physical activity provides a highly visible outlet for the expression of achievement, it is rather surprising that little is known about the achievement needs of older adults, particularly as these needs relate to participation in physical activity (Rotella & Bunker, 1978b).

Notions of achievement motivation seem antithetical to a disengagement perspective on aging (Cumming & Henry, 1961), which suggests that successful adjustments to aging only occur through a mutual and inevitable disassociation of the individual from society. Disengagement theory leads us to believe that either older people have less competitive needs or these needs are directed inward. In addition, as Maehr and Kleiber (1980) have observed, the increased cautiousness and affiliative expressions of older people during task performance may indicate that their motivation to achieve either no longer exists or is directed in new and different ways. Clearly, what is not known is the extent to which older people seek physical activity as an outlet for achievement expression.

An individual's commitment to sport and other achievement-oriented physical activities is dictated by a number of factors, including the intrinsic joy, pleasure, and fun of the activity; the anticipation of extrinsic reward; social evaluation and approval; and the opportunity to demonstrate competence in and mastery of a set of complex skills (Maehr & Kleiber, 1980; Snyder, 1980). It is not surprising, therefore, that many older people, wary of their own physical skill decline, seek other avenues for the expression of their achievement needs. For many people, success, social approval, and fun in physical activity are intricately linked to their abilities to demonstrate physical proficiency and competence. As skill proficiency and the ability to successfully compete decline with age, many people begin to avoid physical activities that enhance failure, loss of esteem, and negative social sanctions. It is unfortunate that, in our Western society, we have not enculturated the value of physical activity as a personal expression of achievement based on intrinsic goal attainment.

Botwinick (1978) suggested that the cautiousness exhibited by older people when asked to perform psychomotor tasks serves as an ego-defense mechanism as they seek to avoid failure, loss, and rejection. Consequently, older people may place greater value on accuracy than on speed during performance (Botwinick, 1978; Welford, 1977a). Older people often avoid responding rather than risking the chance for error. This is particularly evident on complex tasks in which the outcome becomes more uncertain (Botwinick, 1978). Thus, as Kalish (1982) has observed, aging tennis players may begin to play tennis more conservatively and with less enthusiasm, and, consequently, may gradually disengage from tennis.

There are, of course, many examples of elderly athletes who participate in physical activity well into their 70s and 80s. Many of these individuals enjoyed sport and physical activity as children, do not suffer depression or loss of self-esteem when they cannot successfully compete, and may have fewer problems coming to terms with growing older (Winer, 1979). For the most part, however, these individuals are exceptions to the general rule that, with increasing age, most people gradually disengage from sport and physical activity.

Depression and Anxiety

Depression, or deep and pervasive dejection and hopelessness accompanied by feelings of apathy, inferiority, worthlessness, guilt, and loss of self-esteem, is one of the most serious psychiatric problems related to aging (Botwinick, 1978; Butler, 1975; Jarvik, 1975). There are several forms of depression, some of which are thought to have a genetic basis. The peak incidence for depression appears to be between 40 and 65 years; depression is less prevalent after 70 years. Furthermore, depression is more frequent in women than men across the life cycle, although the difference between the sexes is less apparent after 70 years (Jarvik, 1975). Schulz (1982) noted that 21-54 percent of all geriatric hospital admissions are diagnosed as depressed; among nonhospitalized elderly, 2-10 percent are depressed. The incidence of depression among the elderly (as well as other age groups) may have been underestimated, however, because recognizable symptoms are often not diagnosed as being part of a depressive state (Botwinick, 1978).

Depression occurs more frequently in the elderly for a number of reasons. With increasing age, there is greater chance for physical loss, loss of loved ones, loss of occupational identity, loss of income, and social isolation (Botwinick, 1978; Butler & Lewis, 1977; Jarvik, 1975). These potentially tragic changes, coupled with a concomitant loss of pride, self-esteem, and self-respect, make older people particularly vulnerable to experiencing depression.

Symptoms associated with depression include heightened tension and anxiety, weight loss, loss of concentration, altered sleep and eating habits, increased hypochondriasis, psychomotor retardation, and a general decline in personal and social functioning. However, as Jarvik (1975) has noted, it is not known if depression in the elderly qualitatively differs from depression commonly observed in young age groups. Certainly, those who have used elderly subjects in studies on psychomotor slowing should be alert to the potential confounding effects of using subjects who may be depressed (Butler & Lewis, 1977). As I will discuss in Chapter 4, there is some evidence to suggest that exercise has an ameliorative effect on depressed patients and can reduce or eliminate many of the symptoms associated with depression that are common among the elderly.

Anxiety and tension are also major emotional responses to old age (Botwinick, 1978; Butler, 1975; Schulz, 1982). Old people experience guilt and tension as approaching death brings to mind the omissions and commissions of a life once lived. Feelings of impotence and helplessness, and of loss and decline, all demand new modes of adaptation at a time when the aging nervous system is increasingly vulnerable to stress (Butler & Lewis, 1977; Schulz, 1982). Autonomic activity is heightened in the elderly, they are more prone to overactivity, and the inefficiency of previously functional homeostatic feedback mechanisms necessitates more time for the elderly to return to a relaxed state (Schulz, 1982).

It is not surprising, therefore, that when old people are asked to perform a psychomotor task under controlled conditions they often show evidence of psychomotor slowing. Although there is still controversy over the mechanisms and manner by which anxiety inhibits motor performance (e.g., Landers, 1980; Martens, 1977), it is clear that excessive anxiety can cause unnecessary fatigue, distraction, and a general breakdown of central nervous system function. Thus, it is vital that researchers tease out anxiety effects when they examine the effects of aging on psychomotor performance.

Trait theorists categorize anxiety into trait and state components (Spielberger, 1975). Trait anxiety (or anxiety proneness) is viewed as a generalized, somewhat stable predisposition to view life events as potentially stressful. Some would suggest (e.g., Martens, 1977) that competitive physical activity provides a unique arena for the expression of anxiety and, thus, believe that our ability to predict anxious responses during physical activity can be enhanced by examining anxiety proneness specific to competitive physical activity situations (i.e., competitive trait anxiety). Although this may be true, what is more important for the purposes of our discussion is whether trait anxiety remains stable across the life cycle. Biochemical brain changes, tragic loss, life crises, and other factors may lead to potentially dramatic changes in one's proneness toward being anxious. Even if trait anxiety does remain stable, the directions and forms anxiety takes may be susceptible to marked change during the life course. Physical activities, particularly those that accentuate physical prowess, competition, and social evaluation, may be particularly stressful to older people unless proper controls and instruction are provided.

State anxiety has been viewed as transitory feelings of apprehension, worry, and tension, and is often accompanied by heightened autonomic nervous system activity (Spielberger, 1975). Researchers (e.g., Endler, 1977; Endler, Magnusson, Ekehammar, & Okada, 1976) indicate that individuals manifest state anxiety in at least two different modes— somatic and cognitive. Thus, while some individuals experience dryness of mouth, excessive muscular tension, increased respiratory and heart rates, and other symptoms, other individuals become obsessed with negative, self-defeating thoughts but show minimal autonomic activity. This viewpoint (i.e., the multidimensionality of anxiety) is further supported by anxiety treatment therapies that appear to be differentially effective based on the type of state anxiety manifested. What is not known, however, is the extent to which various modes of state anxiety differentially inhibit motor performance. Of equal interest is the important developmental question of whether older people are increasingly susceptible to a particular anxious response, and concomitantly, if older people are more likely to adopt selectively certain defensive mechanisms, such as denial or displacement, in their efforts to cope with anxiety.

Subjective Well-being

Although this discussion of personality changes and emotional responses to aging may leave the reader with a very bleak picture of aging, growing old is not limited to depression, desolation, and despair. Old age is a time for joy as well as sorrow. Older people often show greater sensitivity to the problems of other generations, greater attachments to the family structure, and even capacities for growth and change (Butler, 1975). Many old people have strong nurturing feelings toward the young, evidence enormous curiosity and creativity, and express strong feelings of life satisfaction as they review the richness and diversity of their own lives (Butler & Lewis, 1977).

Thirty years of research on the subjective well-being (or life satisfaction, morale, and adjustment) of older Americans reveals that good health is the most important contributor to positive feelings of general well-being (Larson, 1978). Of course, the desire for good health is universal, but among old people good health is even more important because it means independence and the opportunity to live productive and longer lives (Falk, Falk, & Tomashevich, 1981). Unfortunately, the chances for good health decline with advancing age. More than 86 percent of older people have one or more chronic medical conditions, and their medical expenditures are enormous (Butler, 1975). Frequently, illness and aging are confused as being inseparable, and medical professionals sometimes limit (or even decline) treatment because they view aging as an incurable disease (Falk et al., 1981). Older people are more prone to serious injury and death from falls and other accidents, and they are ravaged by cancer, arthritis, and heart disease. It is no wonder then that perceived feelings of wellness among older adults are so intricately tied to good health.

Research on health and subjective feelings of well-being among older adults has been primarily correlational in design and has most frequently relied on self-report statements (Larson, 1978; Lohmann, 1980). As such, it has been difficult to demonstrate a causal relationship between good health and well-being, particularly when the data are often confounded by variables such as socioeconomic status, educational level, and other factors. In fact, Larson (1978) estimated that the average relationship (or correlation coefficient) in most studies on well-being and good health was in the range of .2–.4; thus, the vast majority of variance on these two variables remains unexplained.

Intricately related to notions of well-being is the self-concept of older adults: their estimates of self-pride, confidence, worth and self-esteem. An important part of the self-concept of older adults (and other age groups) is their body image, or their attitudes toward the aesthetic and functional dimensions of their bodies. Kreitler and Kreitler (1970) claimed that physically inactive older people have distorted body images; they often perceive their bodies to be broader and heavier than they really are. Shephard (1978) contrasted data to show that elderly women have greater discrepancies between their ideal and perceived body image than do elderly men. Distortion of body image produces feelings of clumsiness, anxiety, and insecurity and leads to less interest in (and perhaps fear of) participating in physical activity. This, in turn, leads to further physical deterioration (Harris, 1973; Kreitler & Kreitler, 1970; Shephard, 1978). This vicious cycle also may lead to excessive concerns with bodily function and health (i.e., hypochrondriasis).

The message should be clear. If feelings of well-being and good health are linked, and if good health can be shown to be a function of leading a physically active life-style, than one can logically deduce that physical activity is beneficial to the well-being of older adults. In Chapter 4, we examine this postulate.

SUMMARY

This chapter examined age-related changes in those human functions thought to be intricately related to successful human movement. Changes in cardiorespiratory efficiency, muscular strength and endurance, flexibility, sensory and perceptual processes, neuromuscular integration and control, and personality and emotional responses were examined in relation to age. An information-processing model was adopted to organize data that shed light on the issue of psychomotor slowing with advancing age.

On the surface, the data presented in this chapter seem to suggest that aging is truly a period of decline. However, it is also known that, with advancing age, many people choose to become less physically active. Thus, many of the decrements in physical fitness and psychomotor performance attributed to aging may also be related to inactivity and to the increasingly sedentary life-styles people choose to follow.

The major issue...is not whether these changes occur—they most certainly do—but why they occur, whether their decremental course can be altered, and what implications the changes have for life satisfaction, what coping mechanisms can be most usefully employed, and what efforts others can make to ameliorate the effects of these losses. (Kalish, 1982, p. 28)

REFERENCES

Adrian, M.J. Flexibility in the aging adult. In E.L. Smith & R.C. Serfass (Eds.), *Exercise and aging*. Hillside, N.J.: Enslow, 1981.

Ager, C.L., White, L.W., Mayberry, W.L., Crist, P.A., & Conrad, M.E. Creative aging. *International Journal of Aging and Human Development*, 1981, *14*, 67-75.

Astrand, P-O. Physical performance as a function of age. *Journal of the American Medical Association*, 1968, *205* 105-109.

Astrand, P-O., & Rodahl, K. *Textbook of work physiology* (2nd ed.). New York: McGraw-Hill, 1977.

Atkinson, J.W. (Ed.). *Motives in fantasy, action, and society*. Princeton, N.J.: Van Nostrand, 1958.

Atkinson, J.W., & Feather, N.T. (Eds.). *A theory of achievement motivation*. New York: Wiley, 1966.

Bassey, E.J. Age, inactivity and some physiological responses to exercise. *Gerontology*, 1978, *24*, 66-77.

Birren, J.E. Toward an experimental psychology of aging. *American Psychologist*, 1970, *25*, 124-135.

Birren, J.E. Translations in gerontology—from lab to life. Psychophysiology and speed of response. *American Psychologist*, 1974, *29*, 808-815.

Birren, J.E., Woods, A.M., & Williams, M.V. Behavioral slowing with age: Causes, organization, and consequences. In L.W. Poon (Ed.), *Aging in the 1980s*. Washington, D.C.: American Psychological Association, 1980.

Botwinick, J. Theories of antecedent conditions of speed of responses. In A.T. Welford & J.E. Birren (Eds.), *Behavior, aging, and the nervous system*. Springfield, Ill.: Charles C. Thomas, 1965.

Botwinick, J. Sensory-perceptual factors in reaction time in relation to age. *Journal of Genetic Psychology*, 1972, *121*, 173-177.

Botwinick, J. *Aging and behavior* (2nd ed.). New York: Springer, 1978.

Botwinick, J., & Thompson, L.W. Age differences in reaction time: An artifact? *Gerontologist*, 1968, *8*, 25-28.

Burke, W.E., Tuttle, W.W., Thompson, C.W., Janney, C.D., & Weber, R.J. The relation of grip strength and grip-strength endurance to age. *Journal of Applied Physiology*, 1953 , *5*, 628-630.

Butler, R.N. *Why survive? Being old in America*. New York: Harper & Row, 1975.

Butler, R.N., & Lewis, M.I. *Aging and mental health* (2nd ed.). St. Louis: C.V. Mosby, 1977.

Cerella, J., Poon, L.W., & Williams, D.M. Age and the complexity hypothesis. In L.W. Poon (Ed.), *Aging in the 1980s*. Washington, D.C.: American Psychological Association, 1980.

Clarke, H.H. (Ed.). Exercise and aging. *Physical Fitness Research Digest*, 1977 (Series 7, No. 2), 1-27.

Colavita, F.B. *Sensory changes in the elderly*. Springfield, Ill.: Charles C. Thomas, 1978.

Corso, J.F. Sensory processes and age effects in normal adults. *Journal of Gerontology*, 1971, *26*, 90-105.

Craik, F.I.M. Applications of signal detection theory to studies of aging. In A.T. Welford & J.E. Birren (Eds.), *Decision making and age*. New York: S. Karger, 1969.

Cumming, E., & Henry, W.E. *Growing old: The process of disengagement*. New York: Basic Books, 1961.

Dehn, M.M., & Bruce, R.A. Longitudinal variations in maximal oxygen intake with age and activity. *Journal of Applied Physiology*, 1972, *33*, 805-807.

deVries, H.A. Physiology of physical conditioning for the elderly. In R. Harris & L.J. Frankel (Eds.), *Guide to fitness after 50*. New York: Plenum Press, 1977.

Drinkwater, B.L., Horvath, S.M., & Wells, C.L. Aerobic power of females ages 10 to 68. *Journal of Gerontology*, 1975, *30*, 385-394.

Endler, N.S. The interactional model of anxiety: Some possible implications. In D.M. Landers & R.W. Christina (Eds.), *Psychology of motor behavior and sport 1977*. Champaign, Ill.: Human Kinetics, 1977.

Endler, N.S., Magnusson, D., Ekehammar, B., & Okada, M. The multidimensionality of state and trait anxiety. *Scandinavian Journal of Psychology*, 1976, *17*, 81-96.

Espenschade, A.S., & Eckert, H.M. *Motor development* (2nd ed.). Columbus, Ohio: Charles E. Merrill, 1980.

Etzel, E. Validation of a conceptual model characterizing attention among international rifle shooters. *Journal of Sport Psychology*, 1979, *1*, 281-290.

Falk, G., Falk, V., & Tomashevich, G.V. *Aging in America and other cultures*. Saratoga, Calif.: Century Twenty One, 1981.

Fitts, R.H. Aging and skeletal muscle. In E.L. Smith & R.C. Serfass (Eds.), *Exercise and aging*. Hillside, N.J.: Enslow, 1981.

Gottsdanker, R. Aging and the maintaining of preparation. *Experimental Aging Research*, 1980, *6*, 13-27.

Harris, D.V. *Involvement in sport: A somatopsychic rationale for physical activity*. Philadelphia: Lea & Febiger, 1973.

Harris, R. Fitness and the aging process. In R. Harris & L.J. Frankel (Eds.), *Guide to fitness after 50*. New York: Plenum Press, 1977.

Hasselkus, B.R., & Shambes, G.M. Aging and postural sway in women. *Journal of Gerontology*, 1975, *30*, 661-667.

Hodgson, J.L., & Buskirk, E.R. Physical fitness and age, with emphasis on cardiovascular function in the elderly. *Journal of the American Geriatrics Society*, 1977, *25*, 385-392.

Hoyer, W.J., & Plude, D.J. Attentional and perceptual processes in the study of cognitive aging. In L.W. Poon (Ed.), *Aging in the 1980s*. Washington, D.C.: American Psychological Association, 1980.

Humphrey, L.D. Flexibility. *Journal of Physical Education, Recreation, and Dance*, 1981, *52*, 41-43.

Jarvik, L.F. The aging central nervous system: Clinical aspects. In H. Brody, D. Harman, & J.M. Ordy (Eds.), *Clinical, morphologic, and neurochemical aspects in the aging central nervous system*. New York: Raven Press, 1975.

Kalish, R.A. *Late adulthood: Perspectives on human development* (2nd ed.). Monterey, Calif.: Brooks/Cole, 1982.

Klissouras, V., Pirnay, F., & Petit, J.M. Adaptation to maximal effort: Genetics and age. *Journal of Applied Physiology*, 1973, *35*, 288-293.

72

Fitness, Performance, and Personality

Kreitler, H., & Kreitler, S. Movement and aging: A psychological approach. In D. Brunner & E. Jokl (Eds.), *Physical activity and aging*. Baltimore: University Park Press, 1970.

Lamb, L.E., Johnson, R.L., & Stevens, P.M. Cardiovascular deconditioning during chair rest. *Aerospace Medicine*, 1964, *35*, 646-649.

Landers, D.M. The arousal–performance relationship revisited. *Research Quarterly for Exercise and Sports*, 1980, *51*, 77-90.

Larson, R. Thirty years of research on the subjective well-being of older Americans. *Journal of Gerontology*, 1978, *33*, 109-125.

Lohmann, N. Life satisfaction research in aging: Implications for policy development. In N. Datan & N. Lohmann (Eds.), *Transitions of aging*. New York: Academic Press, 1980.

Loveless, N.E., & Sanford, A.J. Effects of age on the contingent negative variation and preparatory set in a reaction-time task. *Journal of Gerontology*, 1974, *29*, 52-63.

Maehr, M.L. Toward a framework for the cross-cultural study of achievement motivation: McClelland reconsidered and redirected. In M.G. Wade & R. Martens (Eds.), *Psychology of motor behavior and sport*. Urbana, Ill.: Human Kinetics, 1974.

Maehr, M.L., & Kleiber, D.A. The graying of America: Implications for achievement motivation theory and research. In L.J. Fyans, Jr. (Ed.), *Achievement motivation: Recent trends in theory and research*. New York: Plenum Press, 1980.

Markus, E.J. Perceptual field dependence among aged persons. *Perceptual and Motor Skills*, 1971, *33*, 175-178.

Marteniuk, R.G. *Aging, cardiovascular health and human performance capacities*. Paper presented at the XXth World Congress in Sports Medicine, Melbourne, Australia, 1974.

Marteniuk, R.G. *Information processing in motor skills*. New York: Holt, Rinehart & Winston, 1976.

Martens, R. *Sport competition anxiety test*. Champaign, Ill.: Human Kinetics, 1977.

McCarter, R. Effects of age on contraction of mammalian skeletal muscle. In G. Kaldor & W.J. DiBattista (Eds.), *Aging in muscle*. New York: Raven Press, 1978.

McClelland, D.C., Atkinson, J.W., Clark, R.W., & Lowell, E.L. *The achievement motive*. New York: Appleton-Century-Crofts, 1953.

Montoye, H.J., & Lamphiear, D.E. Grip and arm strength in males and females, age 10 to 69. *Research Quarterly*, 1977, *48*, 109-120.

Moore, D.H. A study of age group track and field records to relate age and running speed. *Nature*, 1975, *253*, 264-265.

Mundle, P. Masters records: Men's records. *Runner's World*, 1979, *14*, 88-93.

Nideffer, R.M. *The ethics and practice of applied sport psychology*. Ithaca, N.Y.: Mouvement Publications, 1981.

Noble, C.E. Age, race, and sex in the learning and performance of psychomotor skills. In R.T. Osborne, C.E. Noble, & H. Weyl (Eds.), *Human variation: The biopsychology of age, race, and sex*. New York: Academic Press, 1978.

Overstall, P.W., Exton-Smith, A.N., Imms, F.J., & Johnson, A.L. Falls in the elderly related to postural imbalance. *British Medical Journal*, 1977, *1*, 261-264.

Petrofsky, J.S., Burse, R.L., & Lind, A.R. Comparison of physiological responses of women and men to isometric exercise. *Journal of Applied Physiology*, 1975, *38*, 863-868.

Pfefferbaum, A., Ford, J.M., Roth, W.T., Hopkins, W.F., & Kopell, B.S. Event-related potential changes in healthy aged females. *Electroencephalography and Clinical Neurophysiology*, 1979, *46*, 81-86.

Piscopo, J. Aging and human performance. In E.J. Burke (Ed.), *Exercise, science and fitness*. Ithaca, N.Y.: Mouvement Publications, 1981.

Plowman, S.A., Drinkwater, B.L., & Horvath, S.M. Age and aerobic power in women: A longitudinal study. *Journal of Gerontology*, 1979, *34*, 512-520.

Rahe, R.H., & Arthur, R.J. Swim performance decrement over middle life. *Medicine and Science in Sports*, 1975, *7*, 53-58.

Rotella, R.J., & Bunker, L.K. Field dependence and reaction time in senior tennis players (65 and over). *Perceptual and Motor Skills*, 1978, *46*, 585-586. (a)

Rotella, R.J., & Bunker, L.K. Locus of control and achievement motivation in the active aged (65 and over). *Perceptual and Motor Skills*, 1978, *46*, 1043-1046. (b)

Salthouse, T.A. Speed and age: Multiple rates of age decline. *Experimental Aging Research*, 1976, *2*, 349-359.

Schmidt, R.A. *Motor control and learning*. Champaign, Ill.: Human Kinetics, 1982.

Schulz, R. Emotionality and aging: A theoretical and empirical analysis. *Journal of Gerontology*, 1982, *37*, 42-51.

Serfass, R.C. Physical exercise and the elderly. In G.A. Stull (Ed.), *Encyclopedia of physical education, fitness, and sports: Training, environment, nutrition, and fitness*. Salt Lake City: Brighton, 1980.

Shephard, R.J. *Physical activity and aging*. Chicago: Year Book Medical Publishers, 1978.

Shephard, R.J., & Sidney, K.H. Exercise and aging. In R. Hutton (Ed.), *Exercise and sport science reviews* (Vol. 7). Philadelphia: Franklin Institute Press, 1979.

Shock, N.W., & Norris, A.H. Neuromuscular coordination as a factor in age changes in neuromuscular exercise. In D. Brunner & E. Jokl (Eds.), *Physical activity and aging*. Baltimore: University Park Press, 1970.

Smith, B.H., & Sethi, P.K. Aging and the nervous system. *Geriatrics*, 1975, *30*, 109-115.

Smith, E.L. The interaction of nature and nurture. In E.L. Smith & R.C. Serfass (Eds.), *Exercise and aging*. Hillside, N.J.: Enslow, 1981.

Snyder, E.E. *A reflection on commitment and patterns of disengagement from recreational physical activity*. Paper presented to the North American Society for the Sociology of Sport convention, Denver, 1980.

Spielberger, C.D. The measurement of state and trait anxiety: Conceptual and methodological issues. In L. Levi (Ed.), *Emotions—Their parameters and measurement*. New York: Raven Press, 1975.

Spirduso, W.W. Physical fitness, aging, and psychomotor speed: A review. *Journal of Gerontology*, 1980, *35*, 850-865.

Spirduso, W.W. Fitness status and the aging motor system. In J. Mortimer, F.J. Pirozzolo, & G.B. Maletta (Eds.), *Progress in neurogerontology* (Vol. 3). New York: Praeger, in press.

Stelmach, G.E., & Diewert, G.L. Aging, information processing and fitness. In G. Borg (Ed.), *Physical work and effort.* New York: Pergamon Press, 1977.

Stern, J.A., Oster, P.J., & Newport, K. Reaction time measures, hemispheric specialization, and age. In L.W. Poon (Ed.), *Aging in the 1980s.* Washington, D.C.: American Psychological Assoication, 1980.

Stones, M.J., & Kozma, A. Adult age trends in record running performances. *Experimental Aging Research*, 1980, *6*, 407–416.

Thompson, L.W., Axelrod, S., & Cohen, L.D. Senescence and visual identification of tactual-kinesthetic forms. *Journal of Gerontology*, 1965, *20*, 244–249.

Veroff, J. Social comparison and the development of achievement motivation. In C.P. Smith (Ed.), *Achievement-related motives in children.* New York: Russell Sage Foundation, 1969.

Voight, A.E., Bruce, R.A., Kusumi, F., Pettet, G., Nilson, K., Whitkanack, S., & Tapia, J. Longitudinal variations in maximal-exercise performance of healthy, sedentary middle-aged women. *Journal of Sports Medicine and Physical Fitness*, 1975, *15*, 323–327.

Walsh, D.A., & Thompson, L.W. Age differences in visual sensory memory. *Journal of Gerontology*, 1978, *33*, 383–387.

Weinberg, R.S., & Hunt, V.V. The interrelationships between anxiety, motor performance, and electromyography. *Journal of Motor Behavior*, 1976, *8*, 219–224.

Weiss, A.D. The locus of reaction time change with set, motivation, and age. *Journal of Gerontology*, 1965, *20*, 60–64.

Welford, A.T. The psychological refractory period and the timing of high-speed performance—A review and theory. *British Journal of Psychology*, 1952, *48*, 2–19.

Welford, A.T. Performance, biological mechanisms and age: A theoretical sketch. In A.T. Welford & J.E. Birren (Eds.), *Behavior, aging, and the nervous system.* Springfield, Ill.: Charles C. Thomas, 1965.

Welford, A.T. Age and skill: Motor, intellectual and social. In A.T. Welford & J.E. Birren (Eds.). *Decision making and age.* New York: S. Karger, 1969.

Welford, A.T. Motor performance. In J.E. Birren & K.W. Schaie (Eds.), *Handbook of the psychology of aging.* New York: Van Nostrand Reinhold, 1977. (a)

Welford, A.T. Serial reaction times, continuity of task, single-channel effects, and age. In S. Dornic (Ed.), *Attention and performance VI.* Hillsdale, N.J.: Lawrence Erlbaum, 1977. (b)

Winer, F. The elderly jock and how he got that way. In J.H. Goldstein (Ed.), *Sports, games, and play: Social and psychological viewpoints.* Hillsdale, N.J.: Lawrence Erlbaum, 1979.

Woodruff, D.S., & Kramer, D.A. EEG alpha slowing, refractory period, and reaction time in aging. *Experimental Aging Research*, 1979, *5*, 279–292.

Yerkes, R.M., & Dodson, J.D. The relation of strength of stimulus to rapidity of habit-formation. *Journal of Comparative Neurology of Psychology*, 1908, *18*, 459–482.

4

The Values of Exercise and Practice in the Lives of Older Adults

Lawrence Frankel (1975) wrote:

a twinkly young lady of eighty-two remarked to me, "Mr. Frankel, don't you think that at my age it is rather late to start an exercise program?" I replied, in an attempt to be facetious, "You know that Sara, it was told in the Bible, conceived and bore a son when she was long past eighty." Her reply, which left me with mouth agape, "Well, Mr. Frankel, get me a good man and I will try to emulate Sara." (p. 23)

An outgrowth of our industrialized, increasingly technological Western culture has been the shift from physically taxing to more sedentary occupational and social roles. During the first decades of this century, physical education programs emphasized gymnastics, calisthenics, and other vigorous but routinized activities. Those who were fortunate enough to graduate from high school or college were frequently left with the impression that participating in physical activity was like taking a mustard plaster or drinking castor oil. Consequently, for many people, their entrance into occupational, household, and other social roles seemed to be sufficient in terms of obtaining exercise. As these roles became more sedentary, there was little incentive to turn to other outlets for physical activity and exercise. In fact, participation in recreational forms of physical activity was sometimes viewed as contrary to an ingrained Protestant work ethic. For many people, particularly our old citizenry, there has been little education, motivation, and interest to sustain a physically active life-style.

It is not surprising, therefore, that exercise scientists find it difficult to separate true aging effects from unrecognized disease processes and the deconditioning that results from our increasingly sedentary life-styles (deVries, 1974). I noted earlier that there are striking demonstrations that rapid physical deterioration can take place during even relatively short periods of immobilization. Enforced inactivity frequently produces many symptoms, such as a decline in cardiovascular function and work performance, that are commonly associated with aging (Bassey, 1978;

Serfass, 1980). Thus, there may be some truth to the saying, "Use it or lose it!"

There has been an excessive emphasis on moderation when discussing exercise for the elderly, and an underestimation of what older people can achieve physically. A myth has been perpetrated, without documented scientific evidence, that older people cannot benefit from practice and/or are not interested in learning new motor skills. Physicians and other health professionals have been reluctant to prescribe exercise as an effective therapy for older adults (Butler, 1977–78). As Ryan (1975) observed:

> Rather than encouraging the senior citizen to a life of vigorous activity, our society has tended to push them out of the mainstream and into the backwaters where they drift in a desultory fashion, lapsing into a gradual decline which leads inevitably to a hospital, a convalescent home and eventually to a death which may be untimely. They pay the price with their lives, and society pays in hundreds of millions of dollars for medical and ancillary care services. (p. 61)

In Germany, Japan, and the United States, the belief was that older people, unaccustomed to sport and exercise, would profit little if they became physically active after 40 or 50 years of age (deVries, 1975). It has only been during the last decade that we have come to understand that older people are trainable, and that in spite of the ravages of years of inactivity, we can restore some of the vigor associated with youth. Based on testimonies presented by experts in the fields of cardiology, psychiatry, geriatrics, and exercise physiology before the U.S. Senate Subcommittee on Aging in April 1975, it became apparent that exercise regimens could be developed that were safe and beneficial to older adults. As deVries (1975) noted at that time, the trainability of older people with respect to physical work capacity did not appear to be significantly different from that observed in youth (i.e., the percentage gains were similar); furthermore, these training gains did not seem to depend upon having trained vigorously in youth.

As a result of these testimonies, Congress amended the definition of social services provided by the Older Americans Act to include services designed to enable older persons to attain and maintain physical and mental well-being through programs of regular physical activity and exercise (Clarke, 1977). Subsequently, a number of organizations and programs mushroomed to promote physical activity for older adults. The Alliance Committee on Aging was formed under the auspices of the American Alliance for Health, Physical Education, Recreation, and Dance to promote gerontology and to coordinate and promote programs of physical activity and exercise for the elderly. The committee has worked closely with the National Association for Human Development

(NAHD), which has developed the "Active People Over 60" program in cooperation with the President's Council on Physical Fitness and Sports (PCPFS) (Ostrow, 1980a).

The ultimate goal of physical fitness is to enable people at all ages to live vigorously and healthfully (Harris, 1977). In this chapter, I will examine literature that sheds light on the effects of participation in physical activities and programs of exercise on the physical and mental health of the older adult. Although I will examine the effects of exercise on the fitness stature of the older adult, my primary concern will be the cognitive and emotional health benefits of exercise. In addition, I will review literature on the ability of older people to profit from practice during motor skill performance.

EXERCISE AND PHYSICAL FITNESS

There has been a historical reluctance to characterize the elderly as physically fit and active. Society has come to accept the physical ravages of aging as inevitable in spite of the fact that research suggests that at least 50 percent of this decline may be due to atrophy resulting from inactivity (Smith, 1981). The aging body is viewed as aesthetically distasteful, and yet some of us chide the elderly athlete to act his (or her) age. Thus, it may come as a surprise to learn that the values of physical fitness and activity are not circumscribed by age; exercise physiology investigations reveal that older people can profit from physical training, even if they have been inactive for many years.

The majority of research studies that I will review focus on the effects of carefully controlled exercise regimens on specific dimensions of physical fitness. Naturally, these investigations tend to draw volunteers who may have a propensity toward maintaining a healthful and active life-style. Therefore, we must be careful when extrapolating these results to more sedentary and less motivated older adults. In addition, there may be some question as to whether studies on treadmill or ergometry exercise give us insight into the values of some of the less regimented and vigorous exercise programs to which older people are typically attracted. Finally, keep in mind that dramatic training effects may not be necessary for people to experience the practical benefits of physical activity later in life (Nielsen, 1974).

Cardiorespiratory Efficiency

The majority of investigations on physical fitness and aging have dealt with the cardiorespiratory benefits of physical activity in the exercising older adult. Extensive overviews of the research literature by Hodgson and Buskirk (1977), Shephard and Sidney (1979), and Sidney (1981) suggest that regular performance of endurance-type exercises improves the cardiorespiratory efficiency of older adults. To some extent, this conclusion has been based on correlational, retrospective studies of physically active and inactive men. However, there is also substantial experimental research documenting the cardiorespiratory benefits of regimen exercise among older adults.

Pollock, Miller, and Wilmore (1974) compared 25 male champion American track athletes, aged 40-75, to sedentary and moderately trained subjects of similar ages on several cardiovascular and body composition variables. The data were segmented by four age categories: 40-49, 50-59, 60-69, and 70-75. These cross-sectional data revealed that the athletes' fitness levels were higher than the other groups across age and that pronounced age-related decrements did not occur until after age 60; cardiovascular age-related decrements in the track athletes paralleled the other groups. The authors commented that continuous lifetime training could conceivably retard some of the age-related decrements observed. Longitudinal data (Robinson, Dill, Robinson, Tzankoff, & Wagner, 1976) on male champion runners revealed that although there were declines in $\dot{V}O_{2\,max}$ and maximum heart rate from youth to a mean age of approximately 57 years, these athletes still exhibited superior cardiorespiratory functioning relative to comparable age-related normative (nonathlete) data.

Similar findings were reported for women. For example, Drinkwater, Horvath, and Wells (1975) examined the aerobic power of females, aged 10-68, using a cross-sectional research design. These subjects were categorized into physically fit and physically unfit groups based on their $\dot{V}O_{2\,max}$ data. The results of physiological testing indicated that, across age, the fit women were superior in $\dot{V}O_{2\,max}$ (see Figure 4-1), oxygen debt, and postexercise blood lactate levels. There were no differences across age on maximum heart rate, excess carbon dioxide, and respiratory exchange ratios. The investigators noted that there were sharp decrements on most variables after age 50. Follow-up 6-year longitudinal data on 36 of these subjects (Plowman, Drinkwater, & Horvath, 1979) revealed that declines in $\dot{V}O_{2\,max}$ were similar across fit and unfit groups. However, longitudinal data typically show more accentuated age-related declines than the results obtained from cross-sectional research.

A case study (Faria & Frankel, 1977) was made on a 70-year-old highly trained champion male cyclist. This individual competed in track during college, but 37 years elapsed before he resumed any serious training. At 70, he was cycling 6 miles per day and raced approximately 2,380 miles per year. Tests conducted on resting blood pressure, resting heart rate, maximum heart rate, and $\dot{V}O_{2\,max}$ revealed that this individual's scores were comparable to younger endurance athletes and were significantly better than untrained subjects of a similar age. As the authors observed, however, it is difficult to tease out the relative

80

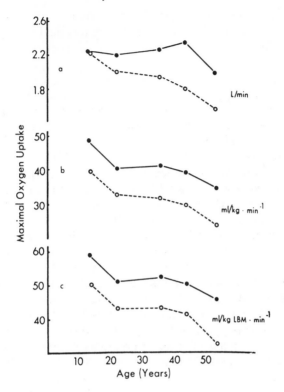

Figure 4-1. Cross-sectional data on maximal aerobic power of females above (●) and below (O) age group means for $\dot{V}O_{2\,max}$. (From Drinkwater, B.L., Horvath, S.M., & Wells, C.L. Aerobic power of females, ages 10 to 68. *Journal of Gerontology*, 1975, *30*, 388. Copyright © 1975 by the Gerontological Society of America. Reprinted by permission.)

contributions of heredity versus early and later training as they impacted on the fitness stature of this subject. Furthermore, retrospective analyses often mask the potential confounding effects of differences in life-style (e.g., cigarette smoking and nutritional patterns), which also may differentiate active from inactive subjects.

Experimental investigations of carefully regulated exercise regimens add further credence to the value of vigorous physical activity across the life cycle. Hodgson and Buskirk (1977) reported that, on the basis of a review of 11 cross-sectional studies of the experimental effects of conditioning regimens, one could expect through training an increase of 16.7 percent in $\dot{V}O_{2\,max}$ at age 30 and an 11.5 percent increase in $\dot{V}O_{2\,max}$ at age 60. They did note, however, that it was difficult to compare these studies because of the lack of uniformity regarding the frequency, intensity, and duration of the exercise programs. Furthermore, the results of short-term exercise among previously inactive subjects may be different from the effects of regular exercise participation throughout life.

Representative of the experimental research on exercise training among older adults is a study by Sidney and Shephard (1978). Volunteer elderly men ($N = 14$) and women $N = 28$), aged 60–83, participated in a 14-week exercise program that consisted mainly of fast walking and jogging; more than one-half of these individuals continued in the program for 1 year. Subjects assigned themselves to one of four groups based on the frequency and intensity of their desired participation. The investigators reported that after 7 weeks, there were gains in predicted $\dot{V}O_{2\,max}$ that were proportional to the frequency and intensity of training. The high frequency–high intensity group showed the most improvement in predicted $\dot{V}O_{2\,max}$, and the low frequency–low intensity group showed no change. Most gains in $\dot{V}O_{2\,max}$ across groups were made in the first 7 weeks of the program (see Figure 4-2). Other evidence of successful training included reductions in body fat and a faster recovery of heart rate following submaximal exercise. Thus, as the authors confirmed, physical fitness can be developed in the elderly, given an appropriate and progressive regimen of exercise.

Studies of the effects of exercise programs on high- or low-fit men (Montgomery & Ismail, 1977) and on institutionalized geriatric mental patients (Clark, Wade, Massey, & Van Dyke, 1975), provided additional evidence that the cardiorespiratory benefits of exercise are not circumscribed by age. Despite the controversy regarding the interaction of training and previous fitness history, there seems to be a consensus that the benefits of training are independent of the gender of the elderly subject (Adams & deVries, 1973; Shephard & Sidney, 1979). Overall, favorable changes in systolic blood pressure, recovery heart rate, blood lactic acid levels, oxygen pulse, and $\dot{V}O_{2\,max}$ have been reported among older adults in response to submaximal exercise. Studies on maximal exertion are more limited (because of the potential hazards of exhaustive exercise), although there is some suggestion (e.g., Benestad, 1965) that changes in $\dot{V}O_{2\,max}$ after strenuous exercise may be more limited among elderly men (Hodgson & Buskirk, 1977; Serfass, 1980; Shephard & Sidney, 1979; Sidney, 1981).

Training modes in most studies have varied considerably by activity type (e.g., walking, jogging, treadmill exercise) as well as by the frequency, intensity, and duration of training. Some studies (e.g., Gutman, Herbert, & Brown, 1977) failed to find a training effect, but serious questions (see Chapter 6) can be raised as to whether some exercise programs for the elderly are really designed to produce an aerobic training effect. The universality of findings on the trainability of

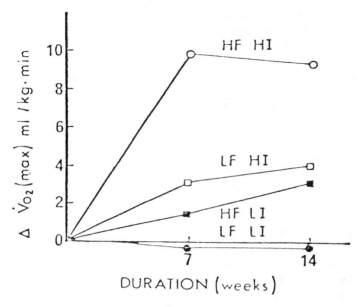

Figure 4-2. Effects of frequency (F) and intensity (I) of effort on changes in predicted aerobic power among elderly subjects (N = 42) after 7 and 14 weeks of training. (From Sidney, K.H., & Shephard, R.J. Frequency and intensity of exercise training for elderly subjects. *Medicine and Science in Sports*, 1978, *10*, 127. Copyright © 1978 by the American College of Sports Medicine. Reprinted by permission.)

older people is apparent when one views confirmatory data reported by Katsuki and Masuda (1969) on Japanese subjects, and by Gore (1972) in her overview of Soviet literature on physical activity and the older Soviet adult.

The extent of physiological improvement with endurance training is related, to some extent, to subject attitude and motivation. It has been suggested by Conrad (1976), for example, that older people exaggerate the risks associated with vigorous activity and underestimate their own abilities. An area that has been given little scientific attention is the older adult's perceptions of exertion during physical performance. In an overview of eight research projects, Bar-Or (1977) concluded that younger subjects had lower ratings of perceived exertion (RPE) than older subjects at a given heart rate during submaximal bicycle ergometry; this difference was less apparent when RPE was examined in relation to percentage of maximum heart rate. In other words, older subjects felt that they were working harder than did younger subjects, when relative work rates were held constant. Bar-Or also reported that correlation coefficients between RPE and heart rate declined with age, possibly suggesting that older adults were less aware of or less accurate in ratings of their exertion levels.

Sidney and Shephard (1977) also found that older subjects had higher RPE scores than did younger subjects, particularly during bicycle ergometry exercise. For a given oxygen intake, they found that RPE scores were more elevated in older subjects; however, RPE ratings were independent of age and gender when oxygen intake was expressed as a percentage of directly measured $\dot{V}O_{2\,max}$. Interestingly, while a 34-week regimen of exercise produced a training effect in the subjects employed by Sidney and Shephard (1977), their RPE scores did not change. Thus, in spite of the fact that these individuals became more physically conditioned, their perceptions of effort did not change during exercise.

Muscular Strength and Endurance

Different muscle groups and individual muscle fibers "age" at different rates. Until the early 1960's, it was thought that training could not improve strength among older people, particularly among those who had been habitually inactive. Recent research studies suggest, however, that significant improvement through training could be expected in muscle function among older adults (Moritani, 1981).

Liemohn (1975) compared the effects of participation in a 6-week isometric training program versus a 6-week varied activity program (balance, coordination, and flexibility exercises) on strength changes in various muscle groups among 52 men ranging in age from 42 to 83 years. Results of the data analyses revealed that there were strength gains among subjects in the isometric training group, and these gains were independent of age or whether one focused on upper-extremity versus lower-extremity muscle groups.

In an interesting, 10-year longitudinal study on physical training reported in the Soviet literature, Deshin (1969) found that a twice-a-week program of physical activity (volleyball, running, balance training, throwing a medicine ball, etc.) improved the number of press-ups and the distance thrown with a 2 kg medicine ball by 6 males and 16 females ranging in age from 51 to 74 years. Information on how the internal validity of the design was maintained over 10 years and on the relative contributions of activity type to strength changes was not available.

Moritani (1981) observed that the trainability of old people does not greatly differ from young or middle-aged people with respect to muscular strength if these age groups are compared on a percentage of change basis. He reported strength data collected on five elderly men (no control group) across an 8-week muscle training program. There was no significant muscle hypertrophy in these individuals, and it was suggested that training-induced increases in the maximal level of muscle activation (i.e., neural factors) accounted for the observed increases in muscle strength.

A number of studies on cardiovascular training in the elderly reported modest or limited gains in strength. Strength gains in the elderly seem to be maximized in programs with specifically targeted strength activities (Shephard & Sidney, 1979). Drug therapy employing anabolic hormone concentrations coupled with exercise has been successfully used to improve strength in the elderly (Osness, 1980). In addition, by the sixth decade of life, strength gains through training appear to be independent of gender (Serfass, 1980). In comparing men to women (or different age groups) on strength changes, it is important to equate these comparison groups in terms of their relative trainability (Shephard, 1978).

Flexibility

Muscles, tendons, and the joint capsules are responsible for movement resistance and, as soft connective tissues, are modifiable through training across age (Munns, 1981). For example, Parks (1979) reported improvements in flexibility among 15 women (aged 65–82) who had participated in a 10-week exercise program that was developed by the NAHD in cooperation with the PCPFS. However, since subjects actually exercised only 15 minutes, three times a week, it is surprising that any changes occurred, unless the subjects exercised on their own. A control group was not employed in the design, making the results somewhat uninterpretable.

Frekany and Leslie (1975) found significant gains in flexibility among 15 female subjects (aged 71–90) who participated in a 7-month program of exercise. Exercise sessions were only twice a week for approximately 30 minutes each. A control group was not employed. Subjects were encouraged to exercise on their own daily. Thus, experimental control in this study was less than desirable.

Kriete (1976) investigated the effects of participation in Frankel's Preventicare exercise program for 7 weeks on specific joint mobilities in healthy females ($N = 27$) over 60 years of age. Fifteen of these individuals were assigned to a control group. The investigator found no significant changes on six of the eight flexibility measurements taken. The exercise program may not, however, have been specific to the types of flexibility measurements evaluated.

Chapman, deVries, and Swezey (1972) examined the effects of an exercise program on finger-joint resistance (stiffness) among 20 young men (aged 15–19) and 20 old men (aged 63–88). The experimental index finger was exercised by lifting weights (attached to a pulley system) for 18 sessions across 6 weeks. Although the old men showed greater finger joint stiffness than the young men, they paralleled the young men in significant improvements in flexibility through training.

Munns (1981) examined the effects of a 12-week exercise-dance program on changes in flexibility among 40 elderly subjects (aged 65–88), one-half of whom were assigned to a control group. Subjects were tested at six body sites using a Leighton flexometer. Multivariate statistical analyses revealed overall flexibility gains through exercise in the experimental group. Because the exercises employed included movements specifically involving the six body sites tested, the investigator also analyzed flexibility changes by body site. All six flexibility comparisons were statistically significant, and the percent changes in joint flexibility as a result of the program are presented in Table 4-1.

It is apparent that the number of studies examining the effects of training on joint flexibility among older adults is limited in both number and quality. Experimental design data gathered without the use of adequate controls are usually meaningless. More data are certainly needed regarding the flexibility benefits of training among older men. In addition, "shotgun" experimental approaches should be avoided. In other words, given the fact that flexibility changes through aging are joint specific, it is incumbent upon us to develop programs that are specifically targeted toward desired flexibility outcomes.

Discussion

The evidence presented in this section suggests that, through physical training, older adults derive physical fitness benefits similar to what might be expected for younger adults. Obviously, however, more data are needed, particularly in the areas of strength and joint flexibility, before optimum training regimens for the older adult can be recommended. Exercises need to be tailored to the fitness needs of the older adult; they should be progressive, carefully monitored, and based on entry fitness levels.

The data I reviewed on RPE confirm that older adults tend to overestimate the strenuousness of physical activity, and thus they may also overestimate the risks involved in physical activity. These factors contribute to the negative attitudes toward physical activity that many older adults have when they first enter physical activity programs, particularly those who have previously led sedentary life-styles. Such attitudes challenge the program leader's ability to advance the psychological tolerance levels of the older participant within a realistic framework of progressive exercises.

EXERCISE AND PSYCHOMOTOR SLOWING

The human brain reaches maximum size and weight at approximately 16-21 years of age and declines about 100 g from 25 to 70 years (Brody, 1970). The brain of a normal young adult contains approximately 10-12 billion neurons, but about 100,000 nerve cells are lost each day. If this decline is linear, we would expect a 15 percent loss in the number of nerve cells from age 20 to age 65 (Harris, 1977). However, the rate of decrease of

Table 4-1

Percent Change in the Range of Joint Motion Following a
12-Week Exercise and Dance Program

Body site	Experimental group	Control group
Neck (flexion/extension)	↑27.8	↓3.6
Shoulder (abduction/adduction)	↑ 8.3	↓5.1
Wrist (flexion/extension)	↑12.8	↓2.3
Hip/Back (flexion/extension)	↑26.9	↓3.7
Knee (flexion/extension)	↑11.6	↓2.7
Ankle (flexion/extension)	↑48.3	↓5.1

Note. From "Effects of Exercise on the Range of Joint Motion in Elderly Subjects" by K. Munns, in *Exercise and aging: The scientific basis* edited by E.L. Smith and R.C. Serfass, Enslow Publishers, Hillside, New Jersey 07205, 1981, $16.95.

nerve cells is thought to be unequal across different regions of the cerebral cortex (Brody, 1970; Harris, 1977), and this loss does not appear to affect intellectual capacity or decision-making abilities as we grow older (Smith, 1981).

Almost 20 years ago, Birren (1965) reviewed literature on health and speed of behavior in the elderly. He concluded that there may be at least two speed factors related to aging: a primary age factor and a factor of cortical integrity influenced by disease, particularly those diseases leading to cell loss and reduced arterial blood flow. As Birren, Woods, and Williams (1980) noted, "although major evidence suggests that slowness of behavior with advancing age occurs as a result of a primary change in the nervous system, environmental differences and disease can interact with this process to modify its appearance and rate of change" (p. 298). Spirduso's (1980, in press) excellent reviews of the literature suggest that exercise, by its trophic effect on the central nervous system, may retard to some extent age-related declines in psychomotor speed and neuromuscular efficiency.

Evidence regarding the impact of exercise and physical activity on age-related declines in psychomotor slowing and neuromuscular efficiency has been, for the most part, circumstantial rather than direct. One line of research has been to contrast, retrospectively, athletes to nonathletes on

87

RT and MT, under the somewhat tenuous assumption that athletes are in better physical condition than nonathletes. For example, Botwinick and Thompson (1968) contrasted elderly men (M age = 74.1 years) to college men (M age = 19.5 years) in a posteriori analyses of RT data. The college men were grouped as either (a) team athletes (or those who exercised regularly) or (b) those who exercised irregularly (or not at all). Results of the data analyses* indicated that although the athletes were significantly faster on RT than the elderly men across trials, there were no differences between the RT scores of the nonathletes and the elderly men. The authors did not, however, tease out the potential confounding effects of fitness versus athletic experience. They suggested that further study was needed clarifying the impact of exercise on age-related changes in the central nervous system.

Spirduso (1980) overviewed data that indicated (in at least 11 studies) that athletes had faster RT scores than nonathletes. It is not clear whether these differences were due to an aerobic training effect, genetic factors, a familiarity with competitive environments, or a combination of these factors (Spirduso, 1980; Spirduso & Clifford, 1978). More importantly, as was apparent from the Botwinick and Thompson (1968) study, we also need data on older athlete–older nonathlete RT scores if we are interested in deciphering retrospective analyses of the impact of physical activity participation on psychomotor slowing.

Studies have also contrasted physically fit to physically unfit individuals on RT and MT. For example, Ohlsson (1977) found that physically fit elderly men (N = 11) were faster than a group of physically unfit elderly men (N = 13) on a paper-and-pencil test of RT. The investigator did not assess the aerobic fitness levels of these individuals, however, because she assumed that there were differences in fitness based on subject self-reports of their previous athletic involvement.

Sherwood and Selder (1979) compared physically fit and sedentary males, ranging in age from 20 to 59 years, on simple and choice RT tasks. Subjects defined as physically fit ran an average of 42 miles per week. The results of the data analyses revealed an increase in RT with advancing age among sedentary males. However, the physically fit group did not evidence any changes in simple or choice RT as the age of subjects in this group increased.

Spirduso (1975) contrasted four groups of 15 male subjects each on simple and choice RT, and their corresponding MTs associated with these conditions. The subjects were grouped by mean age (young = 23.6 years; old = 57.0 years) and physical activity level (based on frequency/duration of participation in racket sports). Overall, the data suggested that the young active subjects were the fastest on these

---

*Had analysis of variance (ANOVA) been employed, there may not have been any reported differences on RT among the three groups.

measures of human performance and the old inactive subjects were the slowest. The old active subjects' performance scores were more similar to the young inactive subjects than to the old inactive subjects.

Spirduso and Clifford (1978) attempted to replicate these findings. However, recognizing that racket-sport involvement is not necessarily correlated with aerobic fitness, they also studied a group of young runners and a group of old runners. Thus, they contrasted six groups of subjects on simple and choice RT and MT. Although age-by-activity interactions were not statistically significant, planned comparisons of simple and choice RT means revealed that the two old active groups were as fast as the young inactive group. (The old racket-sport subjects had lower RT scores than the old runners.) These data are graphically represented in Figure 4-3. Results on MT (arm movement) following both simple and complex reaction indicated that the two older active groups were significantly faster than the young inactive group. Interestingly, activity level was a significant factor in within-subject consistency on RT and MT, but age was not. Old active groups did not show the large degree of performance variability commonly associated with aging.

Similar findings were reported by Clarkson and Kroll (1978) who observed that old (M age = 65.7 years) physically active men were more similar to young (M age = 21.9 years) inactive men than to old (M age = 63.1 years) inactive men in both simple and choice MT (knee extension) responses. Their study is one of the few in which RT was further fractionated into central and peripheral components when looking at fitness differences. These investigators also found that physical activity level, rather than chronological age, was a more important determinant of the effects of practice upon both simple and choice MT responses.

Retrospective studies varying age and physical activity level provide, at best, circumstantial evidence for the notion that physical activity or exercise postpones decrements in neuromuscular function. It is not clear whether sport involvement, aerobic fitness levels, or both are responsible for this apparent postponement. (The Spirduso and Clifford, 1978, data indicated that old racket-sport men still had lower RT scores than the old runners.) The relative contributions of motor practice versus aerobic conditioning on central nervous system function need to be identified and isolated. Confounding variables that also may be related to psychomotor speed, such as motivation, practice, and drug medication, need to be examined.

There have been other lines of circumstantial evidence to suggest that exercise, by its trophic effect on the central nervous system, may retard age-related declines in psychomotor speed. Reviews by Birren and co-workers (1980), Marteniuk (1974), Spirduso (1980, in press), and Stelmach and Diewert (1977) all note that studies on cardiovascularly

89

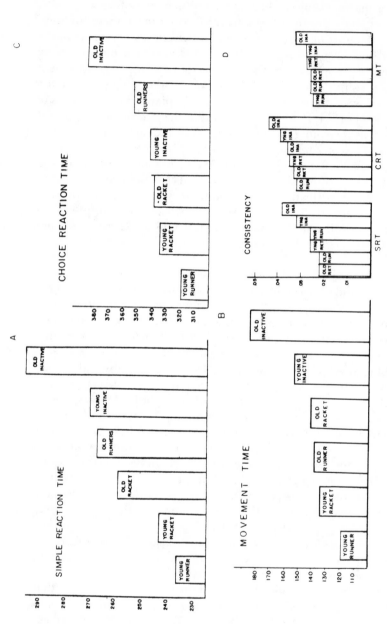

Figure 4-3. Simple and choice RT data among male subjects categorized by age and physical activity levels. (From Spirduso, W.W. Physical fitness, aging, and psychomotor speed: A review. *Journal of Gerontology*, 1980, 35, 854, and based on data in Spirduso, W.W., & Clifford, P. Replication of age and physical activity effects on reaction and movement time. *Journal of Gerontology*, 1978, 33, 26–30. Copyright © 1980 by the Gerontological Society of America. Reprinted by permission.)

impaired men show that these individuals evidence slower RT scores than healthy men of similar ages. Diseases such as arteriosclerosis (hardening of the arteries) and atherosclerosis (buildup of fatty deposits in the walls of the blood vessels) impair oxygen transport to the brain. Thus, decreased cerebral blood circulation and a concomitant diminished supply of oxygen to the central nervous system may lead to reductions in information-processing capabilities. As Stelmach and Diewert (1977) observed:

> In the information processing view, afferent nerves conduct information codes from sensory receptors to the higher brain centers and these centers translate and decode the information contained before issuing an effector command. Accordingly, if the cells of the brain and lower centers are deprived of oxygen these will not function properly and performance will be impaired. (p. 128)

Spirduso (in press) indicated that the decline in cerebral blood flow with age is well documented. Increased aerobic activity could conceivably provide a logical solution to postponing the metabolic impact of a diminished blood supply to the brain. However, the effect and generalizability of exercise on regional blood flow alterations in the brain is unclear (Spirduso, in press). Also, Birren and co-workers (1980) indicated that surprisingly high correlations have been obtained between RT and respiratory function. As I noted earlier, respiratory efficiency can be enhanced through training, even among older adults.

There have been few, if any, experimental investigations testing the potentially ameliorative effects of vigorous exercise on delaying age-related declines in psychomotor speed of response. Boarman (1978) did not find any changes in simple RT or MT among elderly subjects participating in a 5-week, twice a week folk dance program. However, Barry, Steinmetz, Page, and Rodahl (1966) found significant improvements in a ballistic hand speed of movement task among eight elderly subjects (M age = 70 years) who underwent a 3-month physical conditioning program. The designs of these quasi-experimental studies were certainly not conducive to examining intensively the impact of exercise on age changes in psychomotor slowing. Furthermore, these studies employed a limited number of motor performance trials, and the aerobic effects of the training programs employed may have been minimal. Whether one can reverse the deleterious effects of years of habitual inactivity on psychomotor speed among the elderly remains to be seen.

In a more tightly controlled, experimental study on rats, Spirduso and Farrar (1981) reported that treadmill training for 6 months resulted in faster escape and avoidance responses, particularly at shorter conditioned stimulus–unconditioned stimulus intervals, among old trained rats than among a control group of old untrained rats. It is not known if these results from an animal model can be extrapolated to humans. Stelmach and Diewert (1977) reported a personal communication from an investigator who found meaningful increases in information-processing abilities after an extensive training program, particularly in terms of STM. However, published data were not available for review.

Certainly, there is a need for long-term, carefully regulated experimental studies on the role of physical activity or aerobic conditioning in delaying observed age-related decrements in psychomotor speed. Investigators should select subjects who are initially stratified on chronological age, $\dot{V}O_{2\,max}$, and other variables thought to interact with the experimental treatment(s). Learning effects associated with task performance should be minimized (Spirduso & Farrar, 1981).

Besides altering the cardiovascular system, vigorous and habitual exercise is thought to affect other cellular and system mechanisms that are responsible, in part, for increased psychomotor slowing with advancing age. Spirduso (1980, in press) provided the most extensive coverage of these exercise effects, which may be summarized as follows:

1. Exercise retards the age-related decline in the number of muscle fibers, particularly fast-twitch muscle fibers.
2. Exercise provides greater synchronization of motor units and reduces the random firing of neurons.
3. Exercise postpones structural changes in the nerve cell and the loss of dendrites in the aging brain.
4. Exercise maintains hormonal regulatory systems that control, to some extent, the integrity of the nervous system.
5. Exercise delays reductions with aging in the oxidative capacities of the brain and in neurotransmitter substances.

Although most of the evidence on the trophic influences of exercise is indirect, this line of research holds some exciting possibilities for eventually minimizing the impact of aging on human motor performance. As Spirduso (1980) has pointed out, "exercise is a costless, unobtrusive, and self-imposed intervention in the aging process" (p. 862). Thus, the benefits of exercise may transcend the more obvious physical fitness benefits it provides to the elderly. Exercise may also delay inevitable declines in psychomotor speed of response, thereby enhancing the everyday functional movements of the older adult.

PHYSICAL ACTIVITY AND MENTAL HEALTH

In Chapter 3, I suggested that age-related changes in personality and emotion were symptomatic of the joys and sorrows of growing old. Although older adults have the capacity for growth and change and may express positive feelings of life satisfaction, for many individuals growing old is a time of increasing depression, anxiety, desolation, and despair. Functional mobilities decline, and, concomitantly, there are losses in confidence, pride, and estimates of self-worth. This, in turn, leads to an increasing reluctance on the part of the older adult to participate in physical activities where motor inadequacies are mirrored.

Among children and young adults, the evidence suggests that physical activity participation effects both positive and/or negative personality and emotional changes. For example, although competitive sport has the potential to contribute to the moral, social, and emotional development of children (Seefeldt, Gilliam, Blievernicht, & Bruce, 1978), data emanating from some research studies indicate that all may not be well in little league. For many children, participation in little league has been extremely stressful (Ostrow, 1980b; Scanlan & Passer, 1978), leading to burnout and dropout (McPherson, 1978; Orlick & Botterill, 1975). As Albinson's (1975) review of the literature on attitude change and physical activity participation would seem to suggest, one cannot expect favorable attitudes toward physical activity to develop as an inevitable outcome of participation unless the experience is carefully structured to impart positive attitude change.

Data collected on participants in noncompetitive, vigorous physical activities (such as running or swimming) among young and middle-aged adults indicate that these activities may be a source of anxiety and depression reduction, and that they may positively contribute to the overall self-concept of the participant (e.g., Brown, Ramirez, & Taub, 1978; Griest, Klein, Eischens, & Faris, 1978; Higdon, 1978). There has been some debate (e.g., Higdon, 1978; Sachs, 1981) as to whether running, per se, contributes to mental health, or whether the emotional benefits are primarily due to such factors as mastery or the time-outs running provides from everyday, stressful life events. However, it was reported in the *Wall Street Journal* (Yao, 1981) that running may release biochemicals, such as enkephalins and beta-endorphin, that act as chemical messengers, or neurotransmitters, within the brain and spinal cord. These biochemicals, by functioning as "natural opiates," are thought to be responsible, in part, for the so-called runner's high and may also contribute to running addiction (Pargman & Baker, 1980).

Less is known about the impact of physical activity participation on the mental health of the older adult. Anecdotal evidence leads us to believe that participation provides to old people similar personality and emotional benefits that have been acclaimed for younger populations.

For example, Whitehouse (1977) maintained that the psychological benefits to the older adult of achieving physical fitness include the release of tension and aggression, and increased feelings of pride, confidence, and self-discipline. Nicholas (1977) proposed that regular physical activity, in addition to enhancing the older adult's body image, also serves as a release for aggression and tension. Furthermore, he maintained that physically active older people are socially more acceptable. Conrad (1977) suggested that people who exercise look better, feel better, and work better, regardless of age. Cureton (1969), in a secondary, cross-sectional analysis of middle-aged men, concluded that a lack of physical activity and a decline in physical fitness led to a loss of physical courage, increased fears for health and safety, greater tension, and tendencies toward introversion.

Of course, some of these claims are based more on armchair philosophizing than on carefully conducted empirical studies. Some of the claims regarding the benefits of physical activity have not been substantiated among younger populations. For example, competitive physical activities, rather than serving as a catharsis for aggression, may, in fact, provoke aggressive behaviors (e.g., VanDyke, 1980). What are obviously needed are carefully thought-out experimental studies of the impact of physical activity and exercise on the mental health of the older adult.

Wright (1977) examined the effects of participation in a 10-week, twice-a-week physical activity program on the self-concept of elderly females ($N = 90$) assigned to either activity or control groups. The investigator found changes in these individuals' social selves, but not in their personal or physical selves, at the conclusion of the physical activities program. However, the potpourri of physical activities employed (bean bags, balance tasks, etc.) and the limited number of times per week the program was conducted make it difficult to determine why changes in the social self were effected.

Olson (1975) found that a 15-session, 8-week training program of slow stretch, rhythmic breathing, and special upright exercises significantly improved the body image scores of elderly nursing home residents. Similar findings were reported by Sidney and Shephard (1976). Although the training program employed by the latter researchers (i.e., endurance activities for 1 hour/day, 4 days/week, for 14 weeks) was not specifically tailored to effect changes in body image, they reported significant posttest improvements in body image among those elderly subjects classified as high-frequency–high-intensity participants. It has been well documented (e.g., Harris, 1973) that the body image, or one's attitudes toward the aesthetic and functional abilities of one's body, is a very important component of the overall self-concept.

There have been studies on the impact of physical activity

participation on overall personality development. For example, Young and Ismail (1976) studied the effects of a physical fitness program on personality change among young and middle-aged men (N = 90). These individuals were initially classified as young or old and high or low on physical fitness. The program consisted of calisthenics, jogging, and self-selected recreational activities (such as basketball, squash, or swimming) and lasted for 4 months (three 90-minute sessions/week). The Cattell 16 PF, Eysenck's Personality Inventory, and the anxiety scale of the Multiple Affect Adjective Check List were used to assess personality change. The investigators reported that at the end of the program the high-fit men had become more self-sufficient, and all subjects were more socially precise, persistent, and controlled. The investigators emphasized that the personality traits of the unfit subjects did not change dramatically over the 4-month period despite obvious improvements in physical fitness. The hypothesized rationale for expecting multiple personality trait change as a result of this program was not clear.

A similar approach was taken by Penny and Rust (1980), who examined the effects of a 15-week walking-jogging program on personality change among middle-aged females (N = 24) assigned to activity or control groups. Subjects reported feeling better, enjoying more social functions, and not being tired at the end of the day. These statements were apparently not confirmed by posttest score changes on the Minnesota Multiphasic Personality Inventory (MMPI), which suggested that these women did not change in pesonality relative to control subjects as a result of the program. Of course, the use of the MMPI, a personality test constructed on the basis of the performance of patients in various psychiatric diagnostic groupings (Alderman, 1974), would seem questionable in a study of this nature.

Studies examining personality trait change as a result of exercise have also been conducted among elderly subjects. For example, Buccola and Stone (1975) investigated the psychological effects of participation in a 14-week (3 days/week) jogging or cycling program on men aged 60-79, based on Cattell 16 PF score changes. Posttest analysis of data revealed statistically significant improvements on the personality traits of surgency and self-sufficiency among those who elected the jogging treatment. The cycling group did not evidence any personality change. Subject selection of treatment, a 16 percent subject dropout rate, and the question of whether personality trait change could be expected to occur when the time spent at treatment by each individual averaged 114 minutes per week may all limit the potential generalizability of the results obtained.

Bennett, Carmack, and Gardner (1982) examined the effect of an 8-week (two 45-minute sessions/week) exercise program in reducing depression among 38 elderly subjects. These individuals were either residents of a nursing home or participants at a drop-in community senior center. The results of the study led the authors to conclude that a program of balance and flexibility exercises was effective in reducing depression among those individuals ($N = 11$) initially classified as showing signs of clinical depression.

The impact of physical activity and exercise on tension and anxiety reduction among older people has also been examined. Sidney and Shephard (1976) found statistically significant but modest overall declines in manifest anxiety (using Taylor's Manifest Anxiety Scale), particularly among elderly subjects who trained the hardest. In an earlier study, deVries and Adams (1972) contrasted the tranquilizing effect of exercise to the ingestion of meprobamate among 10 individuals, aged 52–70. The investigators reported that 15 minutes of walking at a heart rate of 100 beats/minute was sufficient to induce muscular relaxation that lasted for at least 1 hour following exercise. In fact, these investigators maintained that in a single dose, exercise had a significantly greater tranquilizing effect on the musculature, without any undesirable effects, than did meprobamate. Subsequently, deVries (1974) summarized this line of research as follows: "In the last ten years, we have conducted five different studies on young, middle-aged, and older men and women in which appropriate exercise has been shown to improve the ability to relax both immediately and over a sustained period" (p. 57).

The potential value of physical activity and exercise as a therapeutic adjunct to the emotional well-being of older adults promises to be a double-barreled gain. Not only does physical activity participation offer improvements to aerobic function (and other dimensions of physical fitness), but it also may provide parallel benefits to the mental health of older adults. Unfortunately, the scientific evidence documenting the impact of physical activity on the mental health of older adults is, at best, incomplete.

Some investigators fell into the trap of taking a shotgun approach to the investigation of personality change through physical activity participation. Elderly subjects were tested on a gamut of personality traits, based on personality inventory scores, and the investigator optimistically hoped that at least some traits would show improvement as a result of subject participation in physical activity. The choice of activities for a physical activity program varied from study to study, with no planned, systematic attempt to select physical activities based on their expected, unique contributions to particular mental health outcomes.

Most investigators failed to determine if a training effect resulted from program participation; often, the frequency, intensity, and duration of the physical activity programs cited were quite limited, and thus suspect as to whether they really produced changes in physical fitness. The reader is then left with the difficult question of why, in fact, did personality trait changes occur. Subject expectancies and favorable attitudes toward participation, increased subject attention by the investigator during testing and training, and the desire of the subject to please the investigator are factors that may have confounded some of these studies (Shephard & Sidney, 1979). In addition, theoretical assumptions concerning personality traits suggest that some traits may not have been amenable to change after short-term training. Most important, in order to say that exercise per se, rather than concomitant factors such as mastery or time-out, is directly responsible for certain psychological changes, an aerobic training effect must be observed. In other words, there may be a biochemical prerequisite for inducing selected psychological changes (such as depression reduction) that can only occur after the older adult has engaged in prolonged, intensive aerobic physical activity.

MOTOR LEARNING

One of the more neglected areas in gerontological research relates to the question of whether older people are less capable of achieving skilled performance on motor tasks. In other words, can older people profit from practice in their attempt to learn new motor skills, or "relearn" old motor skills? The absence of literature addressing this question is surprising; perhaps society does not view motor skill acquisition as relevant to the plight of the elderly.

Schmidt (1982) provides an excellent overview of various parameters affecting motor skill acquisition and retention, and the difficulties inherent in measuring true learning effects. He defined motor learning as "a set of processes associated with practice or experience leading to relatively permanent changes in skilled behavior" (p. 438). This definition suggests that understanding the processes or mechanisms underlying skill acquisition is crucial to understanding why motor learning occurs. Sometimes, researchers erroneously believe that changes in motor performance scores are indicative of motor learning. However, because motor learning is not usually directly observable, one can only infer that learning may have occurred on the basis of performance changes. Factors such as growth, motivation, and fatigue may also produce fluctuations in performance that are not relatively permanent, and thus are not usually considered variables that affect learning.

Inferences regarding motor learning are usually based on the employment of *transfer designs*. In a hypothetical experiment, for example, we might be interested in contrasting the effects of varying the post-KR-delay interval* on the acquisition of rotary pursuit skill (a historically popular motor-learning task) among children, young adults, and older adults. The researcher might establish three post-KR-delay intervals, hold the KR-delay interval† constant, and randomly assign subjects from each age group to each of the three post-KR-delay interval conditions (i.e., nine groups would be formed). All subjects would be asked to perform a series of trials on the rotary pursuit test, leading to the possible finding that there are statistically significant performance differences (based on time on target) among the three chronological age groups, particularly at the shortest post-KR-delay interval selected.

To ascertain whether these observed performance differences are relatively permanent (i.e., if motor learning has occurred), the researcher would employ a transfer design. In other words, after a designated period of time, all groups would be asked to perform on the rotary pursuit test under a common level of the independent variable (i.e., the post-KR-delay interval is held constant across the three age groups). The researcher might find that, in spite of switching conditions, there continued to be similar performance differences among the three chronological age groups, particularly among those groups who had initially practiced at the shortest post-KR-delay interval. Thus, the researcher might conclude that learning had occurred; that is, initially observed performance differences were retained during the transfer phase of the experiment.

On the surface, this would seem to be a legitimate experimental paradigm for investigating potential KR-processing differences as a function of chronological age. However, as Schmidt (1982) has cautioned, motor-learning experiments can lead us down a primrose path if they are not carefully designed and thought out. First of all, it is highly possible that the older subjects initially performed more poorly than the younger subjects across all post-KR-delay conditions of the rotary pursuit test. Thus, differences on the transfer test may be due to initial performance differences rather than to changes in the amount learned. It is imperative that systematic sampling differences be controlled, and Schmidt provides several possible solutions to this problem. It is also well known that the amount of transfer between tasks usually depends on their similarity, and is usually quite small unless the tasks are almost identical (Schmidt, 1982). Thus, the selection of a criterion task (to evidence learning) during the transfer phase is crucial. If we had selected a post-KR-delay interval in the transfer phase that had

---

*The post-KR-delay interval is the period of time between the presentation of knowledge of results (KR), or verbalized, postresponse feedback about the movement outcome(s), and the production of the next movement.

†The KR-delay interval is the period of time in which KR is initially delayed after movement.

previously been employed by some of the practice groups, the other groups could be temporarily handicapped until they "adjusted" to the requirements of this new condition. Although there are solutions to this switching problem, they may not be cost effective (Schmidt, 1982). The researcher also needs to consider carefully and to manipulate systematically the rest interval provided prior to the transfer phase, and to equate differences in original learning when examining retention differences across age (Lersten, 1974). Finally, observed differences in learning across chronological age may simply be an artifact of the scoring system employed (Schmidt, 1982); learning under very easy or very difficult conditions may be differentially beneficial to a particular age group.

The research literature on aging and motor skill acquisition is sparse. Wiegand and Ramella (1981) examined the effects of manipulating either the KR-delay interval or the post-KR-delay interval on the acquisition of skill among 60 older adults (M age = 65.6 years) and 60 college-age volunteers (M age = 23.2 years). Subjects performed 20 trials of the Bassin anticipation timer. Generally, the investigators found that the older adults performed more poorly (based on absolute error scores) than the college students throughout the 20 trials. Varying either the KR-delay interval or the post-KR-delay interval did not differentially affect the performance of the two age groups. Even if a transfer design had been used by the investigators, overall initial performance differences needed to be controlled to interpret correctly learning effects.

Surburg (1976) examined the effects of physical and/or mental practice on rotary pursuit performance and retention among two groups of elderly subjects categorized by chronological age (65–79 and 80–100). Subjects from each age group were assigned randomly to one of six practice conditions or to a control group. Practice conditions varied based on the amount of physical practice and/or mental rehearsal of the rotary pursuit task allowed. All subjects were pretested, posttested, and, 8 weeks later, given a retention test on the pursuit rotor. Findings indicated that subjects given the most extensive practice (14 sessions), based on a combination of physical and mental practice, were superior on the posttest, although there were no retention differences across practice groups. However, in terms of absolute values, the younger age group retained the rotary pursuit skill better than did the older age group. Chronological age did not appear to interact with the type of practice allowed.

The majority of studies on motor skill acquisition among the elderly have focused on simple and choice RT and the corresponding MTs associated with these responses. However, most of the tasks employed showed relatively stable performance after a limited number of trials and, thus, may be restricted in the amount of learning required. No studies were found that employed a transfer design when investigating motor learning among the elderly.

In one of the few studies that fractionated RT into premotor RT and motor RT, Clarkson and Kroll (1978) examined the effects of 2 days of practice on simple and choice RT tasks among young and old subjects, categorized as either physically active or inactive. For simple RT (total), only the two older age groups (i.e., the physically inactive and the physically active older subjects) appeared to profit from practice. On choice RT, only the old inactive group failed to improve with practice. These differences are illustrated in Figure 4-4. Changes in both simple and choice RT were accounted for by changes in the premotor component. Significant improvements in MT (in response to kicking a small target following presentation of a visual stimulus) only occurred among the two inactive groups. Physical activity rather than age had a greater effect upon MT, but age was the more important determinant of practice effects in RT performance.

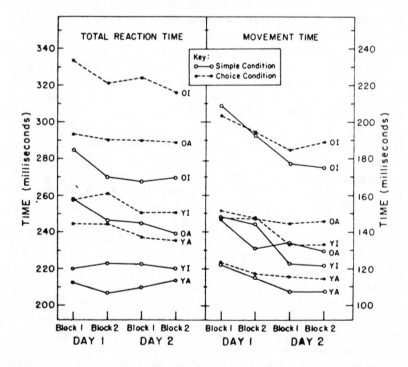

Figure 4-4. Total reaction times and movement times over 2 days for old inactive (OI), old active (OA), young inactive (YI), and young active (YA) subjects. (From Clarkson, P.M., & Kroll, W. Practice effects on fractionated response time related to age and activity level. *Journal of Motor Behavior*, 1978, *10*, 278. Copyright © 1978 by Journal Publishing Affiliates. Reprinted by permission.)

Values of Exercise and Practice

Murrell (1970) examined the effects of extensive practice on changes in simple and choice RT among three female subjects (aged 57, 18, and 17). The author found that although the older subject needed approximately 300 trials before improvement was observed, this individual appeared to gain the most from practice. It has also been found that KR can inhibit the RT performance of older subjects (Hines, 1979). Praise can (at least initially) enhance performance (Lair & Moon, 1972), but monetary incentives did not improve performance among the elderly (Grant, Storandt, & Botwinick, 1978). Furthermore, when initial RT differences were somewhat controlled between young and old, Gottsdanker (1980) found that most old subjects could eventually profit from advance information when getting ready for a response.

Singer (1975) noted that more established and practiced routines may make it difficult for older people to learn new skills. Piscopo (1981) insisted that we do not lose our ability to learn motor skills after 50. Welford (1977) suggested that practice leads to a general convergence among various age groups on motor task performance, although Botwinick (1978) observed that more practice may be required to minimize aging effects as task complexity increases. Unfortunately, there are minimal data, at present, to document these contentions.

Older people seem to require some initial period to adjust to a testing situation before the benefits of practice become apparent. Whether this is due to increased autonomic reactivity, increased cautiousness, or some other factor is not clear at this point. Older people also have more difficulty (at least in terms of verbal learning) amending errors, and they tend to repeat ineffective responses or not respond at all (Botwinick, 1978; Lersten, 1974). It may be that older people have not lost their ability to learn; rather, they may have difficulty unlearning a history deeply ingrained in previous motor skill practice.

SUMMARY

Although there appear to be age-related decrements in most parameters related to human skillful performance, these decrements may also be attributable, in part, to the increasingly sedentary life-style people elect to follow as they grow older. The data overviewed in this chapter indicate that older people can profit from training, particularly training that is progressive, vigorous, and conducted under carefully monitored conditions. Gains have been reported among older men and women on most parameters related to physical fitness, even among individuals who had previously been inactive for many years. Furthermore, the mental health benefits of physical activity and exercise are not circumscribed by age. Reductions in anxiety and depression, and enhancement of the body image and overall self-concept, appear to complement the gains in physical fitness that vigorous physical activity provides to older people.

101

Perhaps one of the more fascinating lines of research is the mounting evidence that aerobic activity may even retard observed age-related decrements in psychomotor speed and neuromuscular efficiency through its trophic effect on the central nervous system. We also observed that the elderly can profit from practice, although clearly, there is a need for carefully conducted studies to document the notion that old people can learn new motor skills and relearn old ones.

The evidence suggests clearly that, while physical activity may not prolong life, it certainly can enrich our lives. It is to be hoped that this evidence will serve as a catalyst for all of us to remain physically active throughout our lives so that future elderly generations will no longer be found languishing in tenement buildings, rest homes, and hospitals.

Has the current generation of older adults heeded this message? In the next chapter, I will explore what is known about the extent of physical activity participation with increasing age, and some of the factors responsible for the apparent decline in physical activity participation among older people.

REFERENCES

Adams, G.M., & deVries, H.A. Physiological effects of an exercise training regimen upon women aged 52 to 79. *Journal of Gerontology*, 1973, *28*, 50-55.

Albinson, J.G. Attitude measurement in physical education: A review and discussion. In B.S. Rushall (Ed.), *The status of psychomotor learning and sport psychology research.* Halifax, Nova Scotia: Sport Science Associates, 1975.

Alderman, R.B. *Psychological behavior in sport.* Philadelphia: W.B. Saunders, 1974.

Bar-Or, O. Age-related changes in exercise perception. In G. Borg (Ed.), *Physical work and effort.* New York: Pergamon Press, 1977.

Barry, A.J., Steinmetz, J.R., Page, H.F., & Rodahl, K. The effects of physical conditioning on older individuals. II. Motor performance and cognitive function. *Journal of Gerontology*, 1966, *21*, 192-199.

Bassey, E.J. Age, inactivity and some physiological responses to exercise. *Gerontology*, 1978, *24*, 66-77.

Benestad, A.M. Trainability of old men. *Acta Medica Scandinavica*, 1965, *178*, 321-327.

Bennett, J., Carmack, M.A., & Gardner, V.J. The effect of a program of physical exercise on depression in older adults. *Physical Educator*, 1982, *39*, 21-24.

Birren, J.E. Age changes in speed of behavior: Its central nature and physiological correlates. In A.T. Welford & J.E. Birren (Eds.), *Behavior, aging, and the nervous system.* Springfield, Ill.: Charles C. Thomas, 1965.

Birren, J.E., Woods, A.M., & Williams, M.V. Behavioral slowing with age: Causes, organization, and consequences. In L.W. Poon (Ed.), *Aging in the 1980s.* Washington, D.C.: American Psychological Association, 1980.

Boarman, A.M. The effect of folk dancing upon reaction time and movement time of senior citizens. *Dissertation Abstract International*, 1978, *38*, 5329-A.

Botwinick, J. *Aging and behavior* (2nd ed.). New York: Springer, 1978.

Botwinick, J., & Thompson, L.W. Age difference in reaction time: An artifact? *Gerontologist*, 1968, *8*, 25-28.

Brody, H. Structural changes in the aging nervous system. In H.T. Blumenthal (Ed.), *The regulatory role of the nervous system in aging.* New York: S. Karger, 1970.

Brown, R.S., Ramirez, D.E., & Taub, J.M. The prescription of exercise for depression. *The Physician and Sportsmedicine*, 1978, *6*(12), 35-45.

Buccola, V.A., & Stone, W.J. Effects of jogging and cycling programs on physiological and personality variables in aged men. *Research Quarterly*, 1975, *46*, 134-138.

Butler, R.N. Public interest report no. 23: Exercise, the neglected therapy. *The International Journal of Aging and Human Development*, 1977-78, *8*, 193-195.

Chapman, E.A., deVries, H.A., & Swezey, R. Joint stiffness: Effects of exercise on young and old men. *Journal of Gerontology*, 1972, *27*, 218-221.

Clark, B.A., Wade, M.G., Massey, B.H., & Van Dyke, R. Response of institutionalized geriatric mental patients to a twelve week program of regular physical activity. *Journal of Gerontology*, 1975, *5*, 565-573.

103

Values of Exercise and Practice

Clarke, H.H. (Ed.). Exercise and aging. *Physical Fitness Research Digest*, 1977, 7, 1-27.

Clarkson, P.M., & Kroll, W. Practice effects on fractionated response time related to age and activity level. *Journal of Motor Behavior*, 1978, 10, 275-286.

Conrad, C.C. When you're young at heart. *Aging*, 1976, 258, 11-13.

Conrad, C.C. Viewpoint: Regular exercise program is beneficial psychologically as well as physically. *Geriatrics*, 1977, 29, 40-44.

Cureton, T.K. *The physiological effects of exercise programs on adults*. Springfield, Ill.: Charles C. Thomas, 1969.

Deshin, D.F. Motor activity and aging. In Muravov (Ed.), *International symposium on muscular activity and ageing*. Kiev, U.S.S.R.: 1969. (*Gerontologia Clinica*, 1972, 14, 78-85.)

deVries, H.A. *Vigor regained*. Englewood Cliffs, N.J.: Prentice-Hall, 1974.

deVries, H.A. In *Testimony on physical fitness for older persons*. Washington, D.C.: National Association for Human Development, 1975.

deVries, H.A., & Adams, G.M. Electromyographic comparison of single doses of exercise and meprobamate as to effects on muscular relaxation. *American Journal of Physical Medicine*, 1972, 3, 130-141.

Drinkwater, B.L., Horvath, S.M., & Wells, C.L. Aerobic power of females, ages 10 to 68. *Journal of Gerontology*, 1975, 30, 385-394.

Faria, I., & Frankel, M. Anthropometric and physiologic profile of a cyclist—age 70. *Medicine and Science in Sports*, 1977, 9, 118-121.

Frankel, L.J. Be alive as long as you live. In V. Simri (Ed.), *Physical exercise and activity for the aging*. Albany, N.Y.: Center for the Study of Aging, 1975.

Frekany, G.A., & Leslie, D.K. Effects of an exercise program on selected flexibility measurements of senior citizens. *Gerontologist*, 1975, 15, 182-183.

Gore, I.Y. Physical activity and ageing—A survey of Soviet literature. *Gerontologia Clinica*, 1972, 14, 78-85.

Gottsdanker, R. Aging and the use of advance probability information. *Journal of Motor Behavior*, 1980, 12, 133-143.

Grant, E.A., Storandt, M., & Botwinick, J. Incentive and practice in the psychomotor performance of the elderly. *Journal of Gerontology*, 1978, 33, 413-415.

Griest, J.H., Klein, M.H., Eischens, R.R., & Faris, J.T. Running out of depression. *The Physician and Sportsmedicine*, 1978, 6(12), 49-56.

Gutman, G.M., Herbert, C.P., & Brown, S.R. Feldenkrais versus conventional exercises for the elderly. *Journal of Gerontology*, 1977, 32, 562-572.

Harris, D.V. *Involvement in sport: A somatopsychic rationale for physical activity*. Philadelphia: Lea & Febiger, 1973.

Harris, R. Fitness and the aging process. In R. Harris & L.J. Frankel (Eds.), *Guide to fitness after 50*. New York: Plenum Press, 1977.

Higdon, H. Can running cure mental illness? *Runner's World*, 1978, 13, 36-39.

Hines, T. Information feedback, reaction time, and error rates in young and old subjects. *Experimental Aging Research*, 1979, 5, 207-215.

Hodgson, J.L., & Buskirk, E.R. Physical fitness and age, with emphasis on cardiovascular function in the elderly. *Journal of the American Geriatrics Society*, 1977, 25, 385-392.

Katsuki, S., & Masuda, M. Physical exercise for persons of middle and elder age in relation to their physical ability. *Journal of Sports Medicine and Physical Fitness*, 1969, *9*, 193–199.

Kriete, M.M. *The effects of a static exercise program upon specific joint mobilities in healthy female senior citizens.* Unpublished master's thesis, Springfield College, 1976.

Lair, C.V., & Moon, W.H. The effects of praise and reproof on the performance of middle-aged and older subjects. *Aging and Human Development*, 1972, *3*, 279–284.

Lersten, K.C. *Some psychological aspects of aging: Implications for teaching and learning.* Paper presented at the Fifth Annual Conference of the Rocky Mountain Educational Research Association, Albuquerque, N.Mex., 1974.

Liemohn, W.P. Strength and aging: An exploratory study. *International Journal of Aging and Human Development*, 1975, *6*, 347–357.

Marteniuk, R.G. *Aging, cardiovascular health and human performance capacities.* Paper presented at the XXth World Congress in Sports Medicine, Melbourne, Australia, 1974.

McPherson, B.D. The child in competitive sports: Influence of the social milieu. In R.A. Magill, M.J. Ash, & F.L. Smoll (Eds.), *Children in sport: A contemporary anthology.* Champaign, Ill.: Human Kinetics, 1978.

Montgomery, D.L., & Ismail, A.H. The effect of a four-month physical fitness program on high and low-fit groups matched for age. *The Journal of Sports Medicine and Physical Fitness*, 1977, *17*, 327–333.

Moritani, T. Training adaptations in the muscles of older men. In E.L. Smith & R.C. Serfass (Eds.), *Exercise and aging.* Hillside, N.J.: Enslow, 1981.

Munns, K. Effects of exercise on the range of joint motion in elderly subjects. In E.L. Smith & R.C. Serfass (Eds.), *Exercise and aging.* Hillside, N.J.: Enslow, 1981.

Murrell, F.H. The effect of extensive practice on age differences in reaction time. *Journal of Gerontology*, 1970, *25*, 268–274.

Nicholas, A. Community program for tension control. In R. Harris & L.J. Frankel (Eds.), *Guide to fitness after 50.* New York: Plenum Press, 1977.

Nielsen, A.B. *Physical activity patterns of senior citizens.* Unpublished master's thesis, University of Alberta, 1974.

Ohlsson, M. An experimental study on physical fitness related to information processing in elderly people. In G. Borg (Ed.), *Physical work and effort.* New York: Pergamon Press, 1977.

Olson, M.I. *The effects of physical activity on the body image of nursing home residents.* Unpublished master's thesis, Springfield College, 1975.

Orlick, T., & Botterill, C. *Every kid can win.* Chicago: Nelson-Hall, 1975.

Osness, W. *Physiological aging and exercise.* Paper presented at the American Alliance for Health, Physical Education, and Recreation annual convention, Detroit, April, 1980.

Ostrow, A.C. Physical activity as it relates to the health of the aged. In N. Datan & N. Lohmann (Eds.), *Transitions of aging.* New York: Academic Press, 1980. (a)

Ostrow, A.C. Some myths surrounding the impact of organized nonschool sport programs on the middle school child. *West Virginia Journal of Physical Education*, 1980, 6–7. (b)

Pargman, D., & Baker, M.C. Running high: Enkephalin indicted. *Journal of Drug Issues*, 1980, *10*, 341-349.

Parks, C.J. *The effects of a physical fitness program on body composition, flexibility, heart rate, blood pressure, and anxiety levels of senior citizens.* Unpublished doctoral dissertation, University of Alabama, 1979.

Penny, G.D., & Rust, J.O. Effect of a walking-jogging program on personality characteristics of middle-aged females. *Journal of Sports Medicine and Physical Fitness*, 1980, *20*, 221-226.

Piscopo, J. Aging and human performance. In E.J. Burke (Ed.), *Exercise, science and fitness.* Ithaca, N.Y.: Mouvement Publications, 1981.

Plowman, S.A., Drinkwater, B.L., & Horvath, S.M. Age and aerobic power in women: A longitudinal study. *Journal of Gerontology*, 1979, *34*, 512-520.

Pollock, M.L., Miller, H.S., & Wilmore, J. Physiological characteristics of champion American track athletes 40 to 75 years of age. *Journal of Gerontology*, 1974, *29*, 645-649.

Robinson, S., Dill, D.B., Robinson, R.D., Tzankoff, S.P., & Wagner, J.A. Physiological aging of champion runners. *Journal of Applied Physiology*, 1976, *41*, 46-51.

Ryan, A. Importance of physical activity for the elderly. In *Testimony on physical fitness for older persons.* Washington, D.C.: National Association for Human Development, 1975.

Sachs, M.L. Running therapy for the depressed client. *Topics in Clinical Nursing*, 1981, *3*, 77-86.

Scanlan, T.K., & Passer, M.W. Anxiety-inducing factors in competitive youth sports. In F.L. Smoll & R.E. Smith (Eds.), *Psychological perspectives in youth sports.* Washington, D.C.: Hemisphere Publishing Corporation, 1978.

Schmidt, R.A. *Motor control and learning.* Champaign, Ill.: Human Kinetics, 1982.

Seefeldt, V.D., Gilliam, T., Blievernicht, D., & Bruce, R. Scope of youth sport programs in the State of Michigan. In F.L. Smoll & R.E. Smith (Eds.), *Psychological perspectives in youth sports.* Washington, D.C.: Hemisphere Publishing Corporation, 1978.

Serfass, R.C. Physical exercise and the elderly. In G.A. Stull (Ed.), *Encyclopedia of physical education, fitness, and sports: Training, environment, nutrition, and fitness.* Salt Lake City: Brighton, 1980.

Shephard, R.J. *Physical activity and aging.* Chicago: Year Book Medical Publishers, 1978.

Shephard, R.J., & Sidney, K.H. Exercise and aging. In R. Hutton (Ed.), *Exercise and sport science reviews* (Vol. 6). Philadelphia: Franklin Institute Press, 1979.

Sherwood, D.E., & Selder, D.J. Cardiorespiratory health, reaction time and aging. *Medicine and Science in Sports*, 1979, *11*, 186-189.

Sidney, K.H. Cardiovascular benefits of physical activity in the exercising aged. In E.L. Smith & R.C. Serfass (Eds.), *Exercise and aging.* Hillside, N.J.: Enslow, 1981.

Sidney, K.H., & Shephard, R.J. Attitudes toward health and physical activity in the elderly: Effects of a physical training program. *Medicine and Science in Sports*, 1976, *8*, 246-252.

Sidney, K.H., & Shephard, R.J. Perception of exertion in the elderly, effects of aging, mode of exercise, and physical training. *Perceptual and Motor Skills*, 1977, *44*, 999-1010.

Sidney, K.H., & Shephard, R.J. Frequency and intensity of exercise training for elderly subjects. *Medicine and Science in Sports*, 1978, *10*, 125-131.

Singer, R.N. *Motor learning and human performance* (2nd ed.). New York: Macmillan, 1975.

Smith, E.L. The interaction of nature and nurture. In E.L. Smith & R.C. Serfass (Eds.), *Exercise and aging*. Hillside, N.J.: Enslow, 1981.

Spirduso, W.W. Reaction and movement time as a function of age and physical activity level. *Journal of Gerontology*, 1975, *30*, 435-440.

Spirduso, W.W. Physical fitness, aging, and psychomotor speed: A review. *Journal of Gerontology*, 1980, *35*, 850-865.

Spirduso, W.W. Fitness status and the aging motor system. In J. Mortimer, F.J. Pirozzolo, & G.B. Maletta (Eds.), *Progress in neurogerontology* (Vol. 3), New York: Praeger, in press.

Spirduso, W.W., & Clifford, P. Replication of age and physical activity effects on reaction and movement time. *Journal of Gerontology*, 1978, *33*, 26-30.

Spirduso, W.W., & Farrar, R.P. Effects of aerobic training on reactive capacity: An animal model. *Journal of Gerontology*, 1981, *36*, 654-662.

Stelmach, G.E., & Diewert, G.L. Aging, information processing and fitness. In G. Borg (Ed.), *Physical work and effort*. New York: Pergamon Press, 1977.

Surburg, P.R. Aging and effect of physical-mental practice upon acquisition and retention of a motor skill. *Journal of Gerontology*, 1976, *31*, 64-67.

VanDyke, R.R. Aggression in sport: Its implications for character-building. *Quest*, 1980, *32*, 201-208.

Welford, A.T. Motor performance. In J.E. Birren & K.W. Schaie (Eds.), *Handbook of the psychology of aging*. New York: Van Nostrand Reinhold, 1977.

Whitehouse, F. Motivation for fitness. In R. Harris & L.J. Frankel (Eds.), *Guide to fitness after 50*. New York: Plenum Press, 1977.

Wiegand, R.L., & Ramella, R. *An examination of psychomotor skill acquisition in relation to information storage and processing capacity among older adults*. Paper presented at the North American Society for the Psychology of Sport and Physical Activity annual convention, Monterey, Calif., 1981.

Wright, A. *An assessment of the effects of a developmental motor activity programme on the self image of aged females*. Unpublished manuscript, Concordia University, 1977.

Yao, M. Loneliness, sure, but have you tried the beta-endorphins? *Wall Street Journal*, December 1, 1981, p. 1.

Young, R.J., & Ismail, A.H. Personality differences of adult men before and after a physical fitness program. *Research Quarterly*, 1976, *47*, 513-519.

5

Declining Physical Activity Participation: A Human Tragedy

A central theme of this book has been that physical activity and programs of exercise are beneficial to our physical and mental health across the life cycle. Yet, in spite of the well-documented and publicized benefits of remaining physically active, there is increasing evidence of a decline in physical activity participation with advancing age. Although there may be an inherent biological tendency among adults toward becoming less physically active with advancing age, this factor alone cannot account for the sedentary life-styles that older people have traditionally followed. In this chapter, I explore several demographic, psychological, and social factors that may also account for this phenomenon.

THE PATTERN OF DECLINE

One of the more universal observations in relation to aging is the tendency to participate in less physical activity, particularly vigorous physical activity, with advancing age. Thus, it is not surprising that gerontologists and exercise scientists have difficulty separating aging effects from disuse or habitual inactivity as they probe the reasons behind the decline in human motor performance with advancing age.

Previously (Ostrow, 1980), I reviewed interview data obtained in 1972 by the Opinion Research Corporation, Princeton, New Jersey, that showed a decline in physical activity participation among 3,875 American men and women with increasing age. These cross-sectional data (see Table 5-1) were from the National Adult Physical Fitness Survey (NAPFS) as reported by Clarke (1974). The data show a marked decline in physical activity participation, particularly vigorous physical activity, with increasing age. Only walking was popular as a form of exercise among these older adults. Very few women of all ages trained with weights or participated in jogging. Thus, activity participation across age appeared to be related to the type of activity in question. Among those individuals over 60 years of age, the most frequent reasons given for not exercising were either medically related or "I'm too old."

109

Table 5-1

Percentage of Individuals in National Adult Physical Fitness Survey Who
Participated in Physical Activity, by Age and Gender

Exercise form	Age group				
	22-29	30-39	40-49	50-59	60+
Men					
	(N = 381)	(N = 319)	(N = 338)	(N = 384)	(N = 517)
Walking	36	27	39	39	46
Bicycling	28	17	18	13	4
Swimming	25	23	15	14	4
Calisthenics	23	13	10	10	5
Jogging	19	8	8	6	2
Weight training	16	6	3	2	1
Women					
	(N = 427)	(N = 363)	(N = 338)	(N = 346)	(N = 462)
Walking	51	45	41	38	33
Bicycling	28	31	20	10	2
Calisthenics	22	17	16	9	6
Swimming	17	16	13	5	4
Jogging	7	5	2	2	0
Weight training	1	1	0	1	0

Note. From "Physical Activity as It Relates to the Health of the Aged" by A.C. Ostrow, in *Transitions of aging* edited by N. Datan and N. Lohmann, Academic Press, New York, 1980; based on data adapted from "National Adult Physical Fitness Survey" by H.H. Clarke (Ed.), *Physical Fitness Research Digest*, 1974, *4*, 1-27. Copyright © 1980 by Academic Press. Reprinted by permission.

The decline in physical activity participation with advancing age appears evident in many industrialized countries. For example, McPherson and Kozlik (1980), in a secondary analysis of data collected on the physical activity patterns of approximately 50,000 Canadians, concluded that the most dramatic declines in participation occurred after the age of 19 and after the age of 64—two points in the life cycle which marked entry and exit from the labor force. It should be noted, however, that participation in some physical activities was defined merely as involvement in activity at least once a year. The investigators noted that the better-educated and more affluent Canadians may have been more inclined to participate in physical activity across age. Data examined by Hobart (1975) on 4,300 Canadians residing in the province of Alberta also revealed dramatic reductions in physical activity participation with increasing age.

A survey by Cullen and Weeks (1978) of the sporting activities and exercise habits of 3,635 subjects (1,683 males; 1,952 females) over 18 years of age who resided in Busselton, Western Australia, during 1975 confirmed that age-related declines in activity participation were not confined to the Northern Hemisphere. Weekly rates of exercise (see Table 5-2) and the number of hours of exercise undertaken per week (see Table 5-3) by this population show a general pattern of declining physical activity participation with advancing age. Interestingly, however, the percentage of people who exercised daily (Table 5-2) appeared to be greatest among those over 70 years of age. The authors concluded that, despite the natural geographical advantages and relatively cheap sporting facilities in the area, most people in Busselton avoided regular exercise.

There have been some studies (e.g., Ludtke, O'Leary, & Wilke, 1979; Palmore, 1968) that have not found a decline in activity participation with increasing age, although other recreational activities (in addition to physical activity) were included in these analyses. For the most part, however, as McPherson's (1978) review of eight research studies confirmed, there appears to be a blatant decline in the frequency with which people engage in physical activity as they grow older. Furthermore, it is apparent that the activities people choose to participate in as they grow older are physically less taxing, as the data in Table 5-1 seem to suggest.

Data collected on 66-year-old citizens ($N = 255$ females; $N = 137$ males) of Jyvaskyla, Finland, in 1972 illustrate (see Figure 5-1) that walking was by far the most prevalent form of exercise for these individuals. Skiing, jogging, and other forms of vigorous physical activity were much less popular (Heikkinen & Kayhty, 1977).

In a more systematic attempt to examine the physical activity patterns of older adults, the 7-day diaries of men ($N = 9$) and women ($N = 11$) over the age of 60 were carefully evaluated (Sidney & Shephard, 1977) prior to their entrance into an endurance training program. Data presented in Table 5-4 categorize their weekly physical activity patterns by either occupational or leisure pursuits. Generally, these individuals spent less than 20 percent of their time in any form of physical activity during work; the most vigorous task reported was stacking books in a university library. Additional data collected on these subjects through ECG tape records and electrochemical integrators indicated that they led inactive life-styles. At different periods of the day, the heart rates of these individuals averaged 70–90 beats/minute, which rarely approached a training threshold.

In a study of an entire community, Montoye (1975) categorized 1,695 males residing in Tecumseh, Michigan, by chronological age and by average energy expenditure per week in active leisure activities. These activities were assigned energy cost values on the basis of established work metabolic/basal metabolic ratios (WMR/BMR). As can be seen in Figure

111

Table 5-2

Weekly Rates of Exercise in the 1975 Busselton, Western Australia, Population

Age (years)	Total no.	Exercised once a week or less	Exercised 2 to 3 times a week	Exercised 4 to 6 times a week	Did not respond	Exercised daily	Did not exercise
Males							
18–19	48	5 (10%)	15 (31%)	6 (13%)	3 (6%)	2 (5%)	17 (35%)
20–29	276	24 (9%)	76 (28%)	21 (7%)	23 (8%)	13 (5%)	119 (43%)
30–39	271	17 (6%)	69 (26%)	20 (7%)	12 (4%)	13 (5%)	140 (52%)
40–49	286	7 (2%)	52 (18%)	20 (7%)	10 (4%)	13 (5%)	184 (64%)
50–59	276	6 (2%)	32 (12%)	17 (6%)	23 (8%)	13 (5%)	185 (67%)
60–69	313	1 (0%)	30 (10%)	19 (6%)	29 (9%)	17 (6%)	217 (69%)
70 and over	213	1 (1%)	18 (8%)	9 (4%)	25 (12%)	21 (10%)	139 (65%)
Total (all ages)	1,638	61 (4%)	292 (17%)	112 (7%)	125 (7%)	92 (5%)	1,001 (60%)
Females							
18–19	48	3 (6%)	13 (27%)	4 (9%)	1 (2%)	2 (4%)	25 (52%)
20–29	324	32 (10%)	90 (28%)	14 (4%)	17 (5%)	17 (5%)	154 (48%)
30–39	329	25 (18%)	77 (23%)	8 (2%)	20 (6%)	9 (3%)	190 (58%)
40–49	334	16 (5%)	50 (15%)	15 (4%)	10 (3%)	13 (4%)	230 (69%)
50–59	366	8 (2%)	40 (11%)	18 (5%)	33 (9%)	23 (6%)	244 (67%)
60–69	335	4 (1%)	33 (10%)	11 (3%)	45 (14%)	13 (4%)	229 (68%)
70 and over	216	2 (1%)	9 (4%)	5 (2%)	22 (10%)	22 (11%)	156 (72%)
Total (all ages)	1,952	90 (5%)	312 (16%)	75 (4%)	148 (7%)	99 (5%)	1,228 (63%)
Total (males and females)	3,635	151 (4%)	604 (17%)	187 (5%)	273 (8%)	191 (5%)	2,229 (61%)

Note. From "Sporting Activities and Exercise Habits of the 1975 Busselton Population" by K.J. Cullen and P.J. Weeks, *The Medical Journal of Australia,* 1978, *1,* 69–71. Copyright © 1978 by the Australasian Medical Publishing Co., Ltd. Reprinted by permission.

112

Table 5-3

Hours of Exercise Per Week in the 1975 Busselton,
Western Australia, Population

Age (years)	Number of people				
	Total no.	Exercised 1 to 5 hours	Exercised 6 to 10 hours	Exercised more than 10 hours	Tried to get out of breath
Males					
18–19	48	13 (27%)	7 (15%)	4 (8%)	4 (8%)
20–29	276	81 (29%)	37 (13%)	11 (4%)	43 (16%)
30–39	271	65 (24%)	33 (12%)	5 (2%)	41 (15%)
40–49	286	49 (17%)	21 (7%)	5 (2%)	23 (8%)
50–59	276	24 (9%)	21 (8%)	9 (3%)	21 (8%)
60–69	313	21 (7%)	34 (11%)	12 (4%)	13 (4%)
70 and over	213	17 (8%)	9 (4%)	5 (2%)	11 (5%)
Total (all ages)	1,683	270 (16%)	162 (10%)	51 (3%)	156 (9%)
Females					
18–19	48	11 (23%)	4 (8%)	1 (2%)	2 (4%)
20–29	324	102 (31%)	32 (10%)	5 (2%)	29 (9%)
30–39	329	81 (25%)	20 (6%)	3 (1%)	25 (8%)
40–49	334	54 (16%)	16 (5%)	1 (0%)	17 (5%)
50–59	366	36 (10%)	24 (7%)	9 (2%)	10 (3%)
60–69	335	31 (9%)	19 (6%)	3 (1%)	14 (4%)
70 and over	216	11 (5%)	6 (3%)	1 (0%)	5 (2%)
Total (all ages)	1,952	326 (17%)	121 (6%)	23 (1%)	102 (5%)

Note. From "Sporting Activities and Exercise Habits of the 1975 Busselton Population" by K.J. Cullen and P.J. Weeks, *The Medical Journal of Australia,* 1978, *1,* 69–71. Copyright© 1978 by the Australasian Medical Publishing Co., Ltd. Reprinted by permission.

5-2, very few males participated regularly in leisure activities requiring a high level of energy expenditure (i.e., WMR/BMR of at least 8). There appeared to be a progressive decline in participation in leisure activities with WMR/BMR values of 4.0 to 7.9 as the chronological age of these subjects increased. Generally, older men participated less frequently in almost all forms of recreational activity than other male members of this community (Cunningham, Montoye, Metzner, & Keller, 1968).

THE CAUSES OF DECLINE

On the surface, the data I have reviewed would seem to suggest that declining participation in physical activity is inherently related to age. Furthermore, it seems that people participate in less vigorous activity as they grow older. However, methodological inconsistencies in the use of designated age and physical activity categories, and extensive reliance on subject self-report, make some of these findings suspect. In addition,

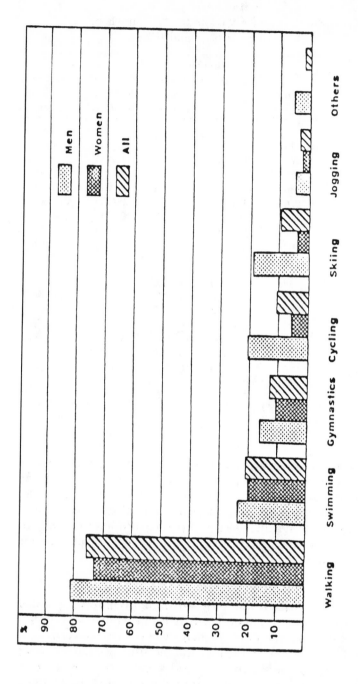

Figure 5-1. Percentage of 66-year-old men ($N = 137$) and women ($N = 255$) residing in Jyvaskyla, Finland, who participated in various physical activities at least once a week. (From Heikkinen, E., & Kayhty, B. Gerontological aspects of physical activity—Motivation of older people in physical training. In R. Harris & L. J. Frankel (Eds.), *Guide to fitness after 50.* New York: Plenum Press, 1977. Copyright © 1977 by Plenum Press. Reprinted by permission.)

114

Table 5-4

Distribution of Activity between Employment and Leisure Hours for 7 Days among Employed Men (N = 9), Employed Women (N = 6), and Retired Women (N = 5) over 60 Years of Age

Activity	Employed[a] men	Employed[b] women	Retired women
Occupational			
Sitting	1,370 ± 182	1,453 ± 194	
Standing	310 ± 60	299 ± 112	
Walking	343 ± 82	222 ± 59	
Moderate physical effort	79 ± 34	183 ± 107	
Heavy physical effort	0	13 ± 13	
Leisure			
Sitting	1,376 ± 93	1,551 ± 226	1,941 ± 247
Standing	332 ± 89	573 ± 216	1,344 ± 401
Walking	426 ± 63	642 ± 167	1,213 ± 258
Driving	437 ± 71	79 ± 65	0
Riding (car/bus/subway)	295 ± 135	216 ± 58	433 ± 168
Bathing/dressing	365 ± 40	386 ± 50	416 ± 69
Eating	720 ± 100	717 ± 160	595 ± 97
Sleeping	3,361 ± 122	3,108 ± 130	3,187 ± 136
Light physical effort	324 ± 81	385 ± 143	548 ± 229
Moderate physical effort	284 ± 91	244 ± 77	264 ± 96
Heavy physical effort	56 ± 35	13 ± 13	129 ± 98
Total minutes	10,080	10,080	10,080
Total minutes active occupation[c]	423 ± 97	418 ± 136	
Total minutes active leisure[c]	1,090 ± 135	1,284 ± 128	2,154 ± 346

Note. From "Activity Patterns of Elderly Men and Women" by K.H. Sidney and R.J. Shephard, *Journal of Gerontology*, 1977, *32*, 25–32. Copyright © 1977 by the Gerontological Society of America. Reprinted by permission.

[a] Employed men worked an average of 5.2 days/week.
[b] Employed women worked an average of 5.0 days/week.
[c] Sum of minutes spent walking and engaged in light to heavy effort.

recognizing that the data I have reviewed are derived from cross-sectional research, it is possible that other factors (some of which may be related to chronological age) are also responsible for increasingly sedentary lifestyles.

Education, Occupation, and Related Factors

Research by Hobart (1975) makes it clear that understanding the factors that differentially contribute to physical activity participation across the life cycle is a complex and difficult undertaking. Hobart examined the relationships of 43 background variables to a derived sports participation

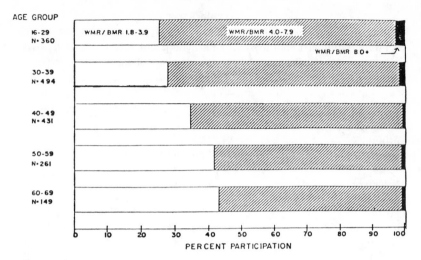

Figure 5-2. Relation of age to participation, at least 1.5 hours/week, in leisure activities of various energy costs. (From Montoye, H.J. *Physical activity and health: An epidemiologic study of an entire community,* © 1975, p. 23. Reprinted by permission of Prentice-Hall, Inc., Englewood Cliffs, N.J.)

index among approximately 3,600 residents* of the Canadian province of Alberta. Although the majority of correlation coefficients obtained indicated that these background variables were significantly related to active sports participation, most relationships, nonetheless, were quite low across chronological age. However, years of schooling did seem to have some bearing on active sports participation, at least among the young and middle-aged men sampled. Interestingly, correlation coefficients of chronological age to active sports participation were quite low.

When examining cross-sectional age data on physical activity participation patterns, it is important to separate cohort differences from true age differences. For example, previous opportunity for participation in physical activity may serve as an important precursor for subsequent involvement, as Hobart's (1975) data suggested. People who grew up and attended school during the early decades of this century did not have excellent physical education programs and facilities (deVries, 1974). Furthermore, there was a lack of scientific awareness as to the benefits of physical fitness. Physical education classes were not coeducational, and there were strict, gender-based rules governing what was considered appropriate physical activity.

Data gathered as part of the NAPFS in 1972 demonstrated distinct

*Females over 55 years of age were excluded from this portion of the data analysis because an insufficient number reported any significant sports participation.

116

differences in previous physical activity opportunity among various cohorts. For example, Table 5-5 illustrates that although the majority of individuals under 40 in this survey had taken physical education while in school, this was true for less than half of those individuals 60 years of age or older (Clarke, 1973). Of course, many older adults have had less formal education than other age brackets, a factor also responsible for the low incidence of enrollment in physical education (Table 5-5). In addition, the percentage of individuals who indicated in this survey that they had competed in school sports was lowest among those over 60 years of age (Clarke, 1974).

Table 5-5

Percentage of Individuals in National Adult Physical Fitness Survey Who Had Taken Physical Education While in School

	% Yes	% No	% Not reported
Sex			
Male	70	29	1
Female	71	28	1
Age Group			
22–29	93	7	0
33–39	89	10	1
40–49	74	25	1
50–59	67	32	1
60 or older	39	58	3
Education			
High school incomplete	45	53	2
High school complete	87	12	1
Some college	93	7	0

Note. Adapted from "National Adult Physical Fitness Survey" by H.H. Clarke (Ed.), *President's Council on Physical Fitness and Sports Newsletter*, 1973, 1-27.

What is the impact of previous education, and opportunity for physical activity in school, on subsequent physical activity involvement? Generally, as can be seen in Table 5-6, the NAPFS corroborated that the more education these individuals had, the more likely was their current participation in exercise. Furthermore, those with more formal education had greater knowledge of the importance of physical fitness and sports participation (Clarke, 1974). It may also be that the more education people have, the more time they have (or choose) for leisure activity. Individuals who had taken physical education in school were more likely to be currently active in noncompetitive sports (Clarke, 1973).

Factors such as occupation, income, and geographical area also impact on the level and direction of physical activity participation

Table 5-6

Percentage of Individuals in National Adult Physical Fitness Survey Who Participated in Physical Activity, by Educational Level

Exercise form	Educational level		
	Less than high school	High school completed	Some college
Men			
Walking	36	34	47
Swimming	7	16	30
Bicycling	9	15	28
Calisthenics	6	11	23
Jogging	3	8	16
Weight training	2	5	10
Women			
Walking	32	46	53
Bicycling	8	22	29
Calisthenics	7	17	23
Swimming	3	13	22
Jogging	2	4	5
Weight training	0	0	1

Note. From "National Adult Physical Fitness Survey" by H.H. Clarke (Ed.), *Physical Fitness Research Digest*, 1974, *4*, 1-27.

118

across the life cycle (Clarke, 1973, 1974; Hobart, 1975; Montoye, 1975). For example, Montoye found that the greatest declines in active leisure participation across age in Tecumseh, Michigan, were among blue-collar workers; white-collar workers (professional and technical, managerial, and clerical and sales) evidenced little change in the number of hours spent at active leisure between the ages of 16 and 59. Although these results may not be generalizable to other communities, the important message seems to be that a complex array of factors present during socialization may be responsible for the increasingly inactive life-styles evident with advancing age. "The decline of activity may be due to job promotion, retirement, social and cultural expectations, lack of opportunities for exercise, institutionalization, accidents or illness, rather than to true biological aging" (Shephard & Sidney, 1979, p. 15). Thus, it may be naive to assume that advancing chronological age, by itself, leads to a gradual disengagement from sport and physical activity.

Psychological and Social Variables

Although factors such as educational opportunities and occupation must be considered, on the whole the evidence points to a pattern of disengagement from physical activity with increasing age. A disengagement perspective on aging tends to blame the aged for their own condition (Levin & Levin, 1980). The decline in physical activity participation with advancing age could be seen as further support for the position that a mutual and inevitable disassociation (disengagement) of the individual from society is a reflection of the individual's successful adjustment to aging. However, studies of successfully aging persons suggest that these individuals characteristically maintain participation in regular and vigorous physical activity (Palmore, 1979; Teague, 1980). Although disengagement is frequently seen as a means of maintaining the functional equilibrium of the social structure, disengagement theorists have failed to examine the complex array of personal and social forces that have created and maintained the conditions under which the elderly live (Levin & Levin, 1980).

Boothby, Tungatt, and Townsend (1981) identified five broad dimensions that they believed accounted, in part, for the termination of sport participation by 244 adults ($N = 134$ females; $N = 110$ males) residing in Great Britain. These five dimensions (based on subject self-report) included declining physical ability, loss of interest, social constraints and commitments, limited access to facilities, and a breakdown of social contacts and networks. Thus, it would seem (as these researchers suggested) that both personal constructs and social linkages may be responsible for increasingly sedentary life-styles. In the remainder of this chapter, I will explore several psychological and social variables that may help us understand why disengagement from physical activity as a function of age appears to be a universal phenomenon, at least within Western, industrialized societies.

Attitudes and Motives

It may be hypothesized that one reason people become more sedentary is because of the increasingly negative attitudes they develop toward physical activity participation. To adequately test this hypothesis, we would have to show not only that attitudes toward physical activity are highly correlated across age with actual participation, but also that we can experimentally manipulate these defined attitudes via actual physical activity participation. Unfortunately, the evidence regarding life cycle changes in attitudes toward physical activity participation is, at best, circumstantial. In fact, much of the evidence is anecdotal in nature.

Kriete (1976) observed that there was a hesitancy on the part of older women to commit themselves to participation in an advertised exercise program. "There was also a noted feeling of resignation on the part of many women that nothing could be done to correct the years of neglect that had ravaged their bodies" (p. 58). It is not surprising that, when subjects in the NAPFS (Clarke, 1973) were asked if they felt they were getting enough exercise, the data suggested that the percentage of subjects responding in the affirmative linearly increased with age. Nielsen (1974) also reported that the majority of older adults he investigated felt they engaged in enough physical activity for people their age.

Conrad (1976), in characterizing older Americans, suggested that they believed their need for exercise diminished and eventually disappeared as they grew older; tended to vastly exaggerate the risks involved in vigorous exercise after middle age; overrated the benefits of light, sporadic exercise; and underrated their own physical abilities and capacities. Conrad's observations indicate that exercise leaders need to be sensitive to the misconceptions and fears regarding physical activity, particularly vigorous physical activity, that many older adults have.

The data on RPE reviewed in Chapter 4 empirically confirmed that, when relative training workloads were equated, many older adults still perceived that they were working harder than did younger subjects sampled. Older subjects evaluated as physically unfit by Sidney and Shephard (1977) prior to their participation in an exercise program also thought they were more active than others of their age group. (Of course, volunteer elderly participants in an exercise program may, in fact, have led more physically active life-styles than the general elderly population from which they were sampled.) It seems that many older adults feel that they are active enough, and fear the consequences of engaging in vigorous physical activity. In Great Britain, Bassey (1978) observed:

There are prevalent social attitudes in this country which militate against even moderate physical activity in the elderly. Vague fears that too much exercise will precipitate injury, catastrophic exhaustion or overt illness bedevil the situation and have fostered disapproval of all but the mildest exertion. The elderly are encouraged to play safe and we suspect that this is to their sorrow. (p. 67)

There are very few research studies that have examined the attitudes of older adults toward physical activity. I am not aware of any studies that have systematically teased out cohort effects in an attempt to isolate better the impact of aging on changes in attitudes toward physical activity across the life span. In fact, in an extensive review of literature by Albinson (1975) on attitude assessment in physical education, only one reported study dealt with an elderly population.

Swanson (1976), using a semantic differential approach, found increasingly more negative attitudes toward physical activity as the age of the respondent increased; males, however, had more positive attitudes toward physical activity than did females across age. Sidney and Shephard (1976), employing Kenyon's (1968b) Attitudes toward Physical Activity scales, found that elderly males ($N = 60$) and females ($N = 64$) placed greater value on physical activity as a form of health and fitness than did high-school students; elderly females were less attracted to the value of physical activity as the pursuit of vertigo than were high-school females; and elderly males placed greater value on physical activity as an aesthetic experience than did high-school males.

I presented a preliminary set of data (Ostrow, 1979, 1980) designed to examine the construct validity of a proposed conceptual model characterizing attitudes of the elderly toward participating in lifetime sports. This model was based on a modification of Kenyon's (1968a, 1968b) conceptual model characterizing attitudes held toward physical activity. Two factors (the aesthetic and ascetic dimensions) of Kenyon's model that I thought (at the time) to be of less relevance to understanding values held for physical activity by the elderly were replaced by two other hypothesized factors: the value of physical activity as a form of achievement expression and as a means of social evaluation. The first new factor was adopted based on a review of literature that suggested that older people may have strong achievement needs that could be channeled through sport and other physical activities. The second new factor was adopted based on Martens's (1976) and Scanlan's (1978) conceptualization of competition as a social process, which suggested that older adults might value physical activity as a means of evaluating their abilities based on information received from other persons vicariously or directly involved in the same competitive process.

121

A 60-item Likert-format attitudinal inventory was constructed, containing 10 items per postulated factor based on a 4-point ordinal scale. The attitudinal target adopted was "lifetime sports," rather than the broader domain of physical activity. Content validity of the questionnaire was established by three judges. Copies of the questionnaire were distributed to 800 elderly subjects residing in a retirement community in New Jersey. Unfortunately, the low return rate (less than 10 percent) made it difficult to interpret the construct validity of the instrument, based on factor analytic techniques. An evaluation of this instrument is ongoing, but I feel strongly that more creative assessment approaches, based on sound linkages between theory and empiricism, are needed if we are to understand attitudes that older adults bring to the realm of physical activity.

There are other lines of evidence we can examine to draw inferences regarding attitudes of older adults toward physical activity. Several research studies have attempted to describe the motives or reasons for older people choosing to participate in physical activity. For example, in the Heikkinen and Kayhty (1977) study on Finnish elderly subjects, it was observed that physical fitness, pleasure, weight regulation, and the preservation of youthfulness were important motives surrounding older adult participation in physical activity. Factors inhibiting participation included disease, lack of interest, and injury or invalidism (see Figure 5-3). The results of a questionnaire administered to 78 elderly subjects ($N = 43$ females; $N = 35$ males) participating in four Golden Age bowling leagues in Calgary, Canada, revealed that their primary reasons for participating in bowling were social in nature: to be with other active people and to belong to a group or team (Gunter & Bratton, 1980). Competition and the challenge of bowling were rated as moderately important. Although the researchers indicated that women valued bowling more for social reasons and less for achievement needs than did men, these comparisons were not statistically evaluated.

The functional impact of attitude change on life cycle declines in physical activity participation is, at this point, unclear. Almost all the studies I have reported have confounded cohort with aging effects. It is highly possible that subsequent generations of older adults, enculturated with a greater understanding of the benefits of remaining physically active, will maintain positive attitudes toward participation. Evidence presented by Sidney and Shephard (1976) suggests that exercise programs have the potential to improve attitudes of the elderly toward physical activity, although Trowbridge (1978) was not able to confirm that exercise training enhanced attitudes toward physical activity among the elderly men ($N = 52$) he examined. (His subjects had highly favorable attitudes toward physical activity prior to participation in the exercise program.)

122

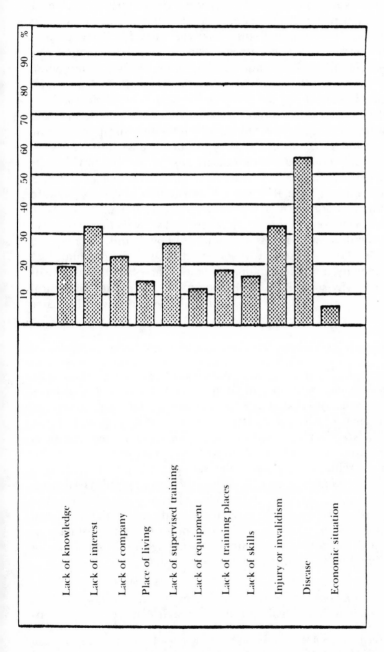

Figure 5-3. Factors inhibiting physical activity participation among 66-year-old men ($N = 137$) and women ($N = 255$) residing in Jyvaskyla, Finland. (From Heikkinen, E., & Kayhty, B. Gerontological aspects of physical activity—Motivation of older people in physical training. In R. Harris & L. J. Frankel (Eds.), *Guide to fitness after 50*. New York: Plenum Press, 1977. Copyright © 1977 by Plenum Press. Reprinted by permission.)

Of course, there is no guarantee that a paper-and-pencil test measure of one's thoughts and feelings toward physical activity will highly correlate with actual behavior. For example, I may think that smoking is dangerous to my health and still smoke cigarettes. Similarly, positive attitudes toward physical activity may not guarantee participation, and vice versa. Nevertheless, an understanding of the hopes and misgivings that many older adults bring to an exercise program is of paramount importance in structuring and promoting programs of physical activity. It would seem logical to expect that a commitment to exercise and other forms of physical activity by older adults is contingent upon effecting positive attitudes toward the values of remaining physically active.

Snyder (1980) noted that commitment to sport and physical activity appeared to be augmented when there was intrinsic enjoyment, pleasure, and fun stemming from the activity; anticipation of extrinsic reward which enhanced pride, power, self-image, and/or health; increased social solidarity and support of significant others; and an avoidance of negative sanctions, failure, and a loss of status. Although this list may not represent the only reasons why older adults remain committed to physical activity, an understanding of some of these factors may give us insight into why some individuals continue to participate in physical activity while others become less inclined to remain physically active with increasing age.

Age Barriers

McPherson (1978) proposed that declines in physical activity participation may stem, in part, from the imposition of social roles, norms, and sanctions that are age related. In other words, age sometimes functions as a socially constructed category defining appropriate role behaviors at specific points in the life cycle. This resultant age grading of behavior may lead to the establishment of normative age criteria for entering and relinquishing select roles, such as participation in physical activity. Unfortunately, this age grading of behavior may also lead to age discrimination or "ageism." McPherson's ideas were the stimulus for a paper I wrote (Ostrow, 1983) expanding on the thesis that a blatant system of age grading may partially account for the relinquishment of physical activity participation with advancing age. In the remainder of this chapter, I will expound some of these ideas.*

Age Stratification Systems. Socialization is viewed as a lifelong process whereby individuals acquire, through complex interactions

---

*For the material on pp. 124-132, I am indebted to Academic Press, Inc., for permission to extract extensively from Ostrow, A.C. Age role stereotyping: Implications for physical activity participation. In G. Rowles & R. Ohta (Eds.), *Aging and milieu: Environmental perspectives on growing old.* New York: Academic Press, 1983.

with members of society, patterns of socially relevant behaviors and experiences that enable them to become and remain effective participants of that society (Kleiber & Kelly, 1980). Through socialization, the individual learns appropriate role behaviors, knowledges, skills, and values. Evidence (e.g., Maddox & Wiley, 1976; Neugarten & Hagestad, 1976) indicates that societies tend to be stratified by age, and that through the process of socialization, age norms form a pervasive network of social control, allocation, and reward.

Riley (1971, 1976) has proposed the thesis that American society is characterized by distinct age strata that dictate the way people behave, think, and relate to one another. "A person's activities, his attitudes toward life, his relationships to his family or work, his biological capacities, and his physical fitness are all conditioned by his position in the age structure of the particular society in which he lives" (Riley, 1976, p. 189). As a result, unfortunately, age inequalities, age segregation, and age conflicts are sometimes perpetuated (Riley & Waring, 1978).

The notion of age stratification systems is based on the premise that age functions as a prime criterion in the assignment of people to opportunities and responsibilities in society. Age strata are viewed as dynamic rather than static and are covariant with respect to the historical events of a given time period (Atchley & Seltzer, 1976). Rapid social change can heighten the differences among age strata, contributing to a sense of uniqueness, isolation, and/or conflict among members of a given stratum (Riley & Waring, 1978). Social mobility of individuals from one stratum to another is universal, unidirectional, and irreversible (Riley, 1971).

Each age cohort, then, can be seen as exposed to a potentially unique set of socially relevant experiences that dictate many behaviors evident across the life cycle, including participation in physical activity. This can be easily illustrated by the recent upsurge in participation in physical activity by women. Until the early 1970's, participation by women in many sports and related physical activities (such as weight lifting) was generally viewed as taboo in our society: participation was viewed as incompatible with the enhancement of the feminine image. Many sports were seen as too strenuous for women, as producing excessive muscular bulk, and as eliciting aggressive and independent behaviors—behaviors traditionally viewed as masculine (Harris, 1973). However, the last decade has witnessed the emergence and acceptance of women in sport, concomitant with the emancipation of women, in general, in society. If one supports a continuity perspective on aging (Atchley, 1971), it can be hypothesized that adolescent females who are active in sport today will maintain a physically active life-style throughout their life course, if they continue to view participating in sport as a satisfying and reinforcing role.

Understanding age strata, therefore, permits us to make tentative

125

hypotheses about the life course of various cohorts. For example, the size of the aged stratum at the turn of the next century should be small relative to future aged cohorts, reflecting the low birth rate during the Depression; however, during the early decades of the coming century, the size of the aged cohort should markedly increase as a result of a "baby boom" that occurred after World War II (Riley, 1971). If one can project the current emphasis on physical fitness across time, then it can be hypothesized that the baby boom cohort will impose great demands for recreational services and sport facilities during their retirement in the next century. Thus, successive age cohorts differing markedly in size may create temporary or permanent disturbances in the social structure (Riley & Waring, 1978).

Clearly, however, the use of chronological age alone as a predictor of human behavior and events is inadequate. It is naive to make judgments about physical (and mental) functioning on the basis of age without considering the social context in which these judgments are made. It is Neugarten's contention (Neugarten, 1980; Neugarten & Datan, 1973; Neugarten & Hagestad, 1976) that life time and historical time must be examined within the framework of social time: that is, within the context of understanding how age roles, age norms, and age statuses systematically regulate self-perceptions and human behavior.

Age Roles and Age Norms. In West Virginia, the Monongalia County Consolidated Recreation Commission sponsored an Over the Hump Basketball League for individuals over 30 years of age. Until 2 years ago, one of the modified basketball rules in this league specified that no fast breaks were allowed (i.e., the offensive team could not bring the ball down until the defensive team had a chance to set themselves up at their end of the court). Pete Rose, the professional baseball player, was characterized as the "ageless wonder" by an Associated Press writer as he approached the National League hitting record at the ripe old age (in baseball) of 41. The Three-Quarter Century Softball Club, formed around 1930 in St. Petersburg, Florida, initially prohibited base running to prevent participants from "dying on the bases" (Kaplan, 1979). During the 1970's, George Allen, coach of the Washington Redskins professional football team, recruited experienced defensive linemen and linebackers in their 30s; they were known as the Over-the-Hill Gang. The United States Handball Association (as do other sport associations) stratify individuals by age when setting up tournaments; the Masters Handball tournaments are for individuals over 40, and the Golden Masters tournaments are for individuals over 50.

These examples serve to illustrate that age, like race or sex, is an attribute that clearly regulates many of the normative expectations affecting participation in sport and physical activity. Age-related norms

126

tell us that children go to school, adults get married, and the elderly should not be interested in sex or in singles in tennis. Neugarten and Datan (1973) indicated that different sets of age expectations and age statuses operate across and within societies. "Every society has a system of social expectations regarding age-appropriate behavior, and these expectations are internalized as the individual grows up and grows old, and as he moves from one age stratum to the next" (Neugarten & Datan, 1973, p. 59). Through socialization, individual members of each cohort learn specific roles based on age, and the concomitant behaviors associated with each of these roles (Neugarten & Hagestad, 1976).

Problems of aging are magnified during life course transitions when the individual must relinquish old roles and adjust to new ones (Riley & Waring, 1978). For example, Botwinick (1978) noted that sex roles sometimes reverse during old age—women become more tolerant of their aggressive impulses, and men become more nurturant and affiliative. As Botwinick speculated, loss of the male work role, and the rebellion of (some) women against a lifelong history of dependence and submissiveness may account for this role reversal.

Conceptually, a system of age grading produces at least two forms of age-appropriate behavior: *ascriptive* age norms and *consensual* age norms (Neugarten & Datan, 1973). Ascriptive age norms are based on clearly specified, societal, age-regulated rules and constraints. For example, in many states it is illegal to drive a car before 16 and to drink alcoholic beverages before 18 years of age; mandatory retirement laws dictate retirement at age 70. In sport, entries into tournaments are usually stratified according to chronological age. Unfortunately, ascriptive age norms lead to age segregation, age inequalities, and conflict. For example, old people in retirement communities are sometimes isolated from younger friends and relatives, although Botwinick (1978) felt that age-segregated rather than age-integrated communities may be better off because of shared cohort experiences.

Consensual age norms specify the assumed age range in which people are expected to acquire or relinquish certain roles. For example, some people may make fun of dating or sexual activities among the elderly. Also, there are few cases of "dirty old men" (Calderone, 1978). In sport and physical activity, it is often assumed that one will retreat from singles to doubles in handball or tennis with advancing age. The playing of touch football would probably be viewed as childish for middle-aged men (and as abhorrent for middle-aged women). In fact, the promotion of "lifetime" sports suggests the differential acceptability of participating in various sports at specific points in the life cycle. Pasini (1975) suggested that sports requiring strength, rapidity of movements, and quick reactions should be contraindicated in old age. Pullias (1977) maintained that activities centered on physical prowess and bodily skill run the risk of being viewed by the elderly as empty, artificial, and even repugnant.

In short, consensual age norms lead each of us to develop built-in time clocks that carefully regulate the roles we assume when we are on time and relinquish when we are off time. Our sensitivity to this time clock influences our pride and estimates of self-worth (Neugarten & Datan, 1973). How many of us have enhanced (or protected) our self-esteem in sport by proclaiming, "Take it easy on the old man"? As Ellfeldt and Lowman (1973) observed, it is easy to declare that sport and exercise are for young people, and that acting your age means sitting quietly or shuffling along slowly and carefully for short distances.

This is not to suggest that gender, race, education, opportunity, affluence, and other factors do not mitigate involvement in sport and physical activity. Rather, I contend that people have underestimated the extent to which age-regulated social networks form a pervasive system of control, allocation, and reward in sport.

Ageism. In ancient Roman times, Cicero characterized the physical activity needs of old age as follows:

> Let others, then, have their weapons, their horses and their spears, their fencing-foils, and games of ball, their swimming contests and foot-races, and out of many sports leave us old fellows our dice and knuckle-bones. Or take away the dice-box, too, if you will, since old age can be happy without it. (Falconer, trans., 1964, p. 71)

Age role stereotypes refer to a set of commonly held beliefs about the way people are supposed to behave based on age. For example, old age is typically characterized as a time of isolation, poverty, and sickness. The older person is traditionally viewed as someone who moves and thinks slowly, who lacks creativity and ambition, and who is irritable, cantankerous, shallow, crazy, rigid, conservative, and enfeebled—in short, the picture of physical and mental decline (Butler, 1975). As Comfort (1978) noted, however, "old people become crazy for three reasons—because they were crazy when young, because they have an illness, or because we drive them crazy" (p. 79).

When our views about aging are discriminatory and prejudicial in nature, we are guilty of practicing ageism (Butler, 1969). Trippatt (1980), in a recent essay on ageism in *Time,* warned that the foreclosure of the elderly from society's respect and admiration will mean serious generational conflict in the future. Butler (1969) prophesized that ageism would parallel racism as the great issue of the remaining decades of this century. In fact, there are analogies between racism and ageism, as Maggie Kuhn (1978), leader of the Gray Panthers, noted:

1. Both are responses of our society to individuals and groups considered inferior.
2. Both deprive certain individuals and groups of status and the right to control their own destinies.
3. Both result in social and economic discrimination and deprivation.
4. Both deprive society of the contributions of many competent, gifted, and creative people.
5. Both result in alienation, despair, and hostility.

The practice of ageism is rampant in our society. Perhaps the most visible example is the picture of older adults seen in advertising. Usually, they are seen as decrepit and toothless consumers of laxatives, denture adhesives, or sleeping pills. Most television commercials lead us to believe that fun and vigorous leisure activity belong solely to the young. How often have we seen a physically active older adult portrayed on television? Advertisers are beginning to recognize, however, that the older segment of our population is more diverse than homogeneous and is growing in importance. "It is becoming increasingly inaccurate to stereotype the elderly as sedentary and nonresponsive to life style changes" (Smith & Serfass, 1981, p. 9). As the *Wall Street Journal* (Abrams, 1981) pointed out, older adults drink Pepsi, too.

A Louis Harris & Associates, Inc., survey (1978) of 4,254 Americans in 1974 on the myths and realities of growing old found that older people did not see themselves as destitute, lonely, or in poor health to the degree young people saw them. Nor did they see themselves as "aged." However, most old people were not seen in this survey as active, efficient, or alert by those classified as young. Only 41 percent of the young considered old people very physically active.

In sport and physical activity, the practice of ageism is often less visible and apparent. There is an underlying assumption of declining reaction and movement speed and an overall reduction in physical function with increasing age. Opportunities and incentives for continued practice of proficiently executed motor skills diminish. The individual develops reduced expectancies for cardiovascular and psychomotor function. These diminished self-expectancies, coupled with social expectations that one should act his/her age and that one should be less competitive and expect less from a competitive outcome, lead many individuals to disengage gradually from sport and physical activity as they grow older. Winer (1979) discussed this phenomenon with reference to the elderly "jock":

The elderly jock, whatever his earlier competence, can no longer confidently regard himself as a good player, but must accept himself

129

as "good for my age," and then as time goes on, take consolation in still playing hard, and then finally find solace in managing to play at all. Period. If he cannot accept, respect and feel pride even as his abilities diminish, he will dropout, becoming an ex-jock, instead of being an elderly one. (p. 197)

Ageism is also evident in the blatant misuse of chronological age as the sole criterion for determining entry levels in competitive sport tournaments. Why have physical educators not considered developmental function, as well as age, in assigning people to competitive slots? Although there may be inevitable decrements in psychomotor function with advancing age, we cannot underestimate disuse and inactivity as factors contributing to this decline. Age matching has not been shown to be effective in youth sports, and we should not expect better results at later points in the life cycle.

Unfortunately, the empirical evidence shedding light on the phenomena of ageism and the age grading of sport and physical activity is nonexistent. This is particularly surprising in view of the enormous attention devoted to racism and sexism in sport, which has paralleled, in general, society's increasing concerns with these social issues. Although several authors (e.g., McPherson, 1978; McPherson & Kozlik, 1980; Snyder, 1980) have discussed the potential impact of ageism, age norms, and age stratification systems on participation in physical activity, carefully designed empirical investigations of these phenomena would appear warranted.

Some Preliminary Data. My colleagues and I (Ostrow, Jones, & Spiker, 1981; Ostrow & Spiker, 1981) have initiated a set of investigations designed to examine and contrast the typing of sport participation based on age role and/or sex role appropriateness. Research (e.g., Jones, 1979; Lewko & Greendorfer, 1978) on sex role stereotyping has disclosed that attitudes toward participation in sport are based, to some extent, on gender appropriateness. Of interest was the extent to which sport participation would be viewed as differentially acceptable based on age role or sex role appropriateness.

Samples of 93 undergraduate female nursing students (Ostrow et al., 1981; Study 1) and 444 students (Ostrow & Spiker, 1981; Study 2) enrolled in the physical education basic instructional program at West Virginia University were administered an Activity Appropriateness Scale (AAS; Figure 5-4) developed by the investigators and Bem's (1974) Sex Role Inventory. Subjects were asked to rate on the AAS how appropriate they felt it was for eight referent persons, who varied in assigned chronological age (20, 40, 60, or 80) and assigned gender, to participate in 12 designated physical activities, including bowling, ballet, tennis, the shot put, basketball, swimming, and bicycling. These 12 activities

Declining Physical Activity

ACTIVITY APPROPRIATENESS SCALE

DIRECTIONS: Below are described eight (8) different individuals. In addition, a list of twelve (12) different sport activities is provided. Please rate how appropriate you feel it is for each individual listed to participate in each activity using the following scale:

1 – VERY INAPPROPRIATE
2 – INAPPROPRIATE
3 – SOMEWHAT INAPPROPRIATE
4 – NEUTRAL FEELINGS
5 – SOMEWHAT APPROPRIATE
6 – APPROPRIATE
7 – VERY APPROPRIATE

EXAMPLE

	Tennis	Basketball	Jogging	Racquetball	Figure Skating	Bicycling	Archery	Marathon Race	Swimming	Bowling	Shot Put	Ballet
15 YEAR OLD HEALTHY MALE	6	6	7	ETC.		ETC.			ETC.		ETC.	

PLEASE RATE FOR THE FOLLOWING INDIVIDUALS

1. 20 YEAR OLD HEALTHY FEMALE
2. 80 YEAR OLD HEALTHY FEMALE
3. 40 YEAR OLD HEALTHY FEMALE
4. 60 YEAR OLD HEALTHY MALE
5. 20 YEAR OLD HEALTHY MALE
6. 60 YEAR OLD HEALTHY FEMALE
7. 40 YEAR OLD HEALTHY MALE
8. 80 YEAR OLD HEALTHY MALE

Figure 5-4. An AAS to assess the typing of sport participation based on age role and/or sex role appropriateness.

131

were selected based on a literature review that identified certain physical activities as being stereotyped more masculine or feminine (Del Rey, 1976; Fisher, Genovese, Morris, & Morris, 1978) and suggested that certain physical activities may be viewed as differentially appropriate at specific points in the life cycle (e.g. Pasini, 1975). The order of presentation of the eight referent persons and 12 physical activities was randomly assigned on the AAS.

The data from both investigations were analyzed using both univariate and multivariate ANOVA. The results of the studies were remarkably consistent. With respect to the typing of sport participation based on age appropriateness, these subjects viewed participation in each activity as less appropriate as the assigned age of the referent person increased from 20 to 40 to 60 to 80. The main effect of age of the referent person accounted for an average of 27.99 and 28.28 percent of the variance of subjects' responses to the AAS in Study 1 and Study 2, respectively. The variance estimates accounted for by age for each physical activity were remarkably consistent across both investigations. Age-regulated social prescriptions appeared to be more evident for basketball, tennis, and racquetball than for bowling or archery. Accountable variance estimates for gender typing (Study 1 = 1.45 percent; Study 2 = 2.97 percent) were small.

The results of both investigations provided evidence that age is a far more potent attribute than gender in dictating these individuals' perceptions of the appropriateness of participating in physical activity across the life cycle. Clearly, the age grading of physical activity must be verified among a number of cohorts (besides college students). Will older adults of similar background view older adult participation as more acceptable? Of particular interest is the important developmental question of when and how age role expectancies for physical activity participation first evolve. Young children seem to have clear social prescriptions for what older persons can and cannot do (McTavish, 1971). How important are physically active parents and grandparents as role models for our children? What impact has television had in portraying the older adult as listless and decrepit, rather than as active and alive?

Recently, Neugarten (1980) optimistically predicted that we were on the verge of becoming an age-irrelevant society—that the internal age-regulated time clock she used to write about was no longer as powerful or as compelling. It appears that her message had not yet reached the college students we surveyed. They had clear, age-regulated social prescriptions regarding the extent to which people should be involved in physical activity as they grow older.

SUMMARY

In this chapter, I presented evidence that appears to document a decline in physical activity participation with advancing age, at least within Western, industrialized societies. However, the confounding effects of cohort differences rule out the conclusion, at least for now, that increasingly sedentary life-styles are inevitable manifestations of the aging process. Differences in education, opportunity, and affluence may also be responsible for the observed decline in physical activity participation with advancing age.

I also examined some psychological and social factors behind the gradual disengagement from physical activity. Excessive fears of vigorous activity, an underestimation by the elderly of their own physical abilities and capacities, and social expectancies that one should be less physically active as one grows older all contribute to negative attitudes, lack of commitment, and a universal, age-related "turn-off" from physical activity participation. The stratification of society by age and the concomitant development of age roles, age norms, and age statuses were postulated as also contributing to increasingly sedentary life-styles with advancing age. Preliminary data were presented that suggested that age typing was a prominent factor in characterizing what is appropriate and inappropriate physical activity participation across the life cycle.

It would be fallacious to assume that the age grading of human behavior can account for the myriad of variables that preclude involvement in sport and physical activity with advancing age. Similarly, it would be fallacious to promote vigorous physical activity participation for all adults without first adapting and prescribing physical activities based on individual tolerance levels. In Chapter 6, I will explore a number of important principles to consider when programming physical activities for the older adult. It should be clear, however, that participation in physical activity must be based on developmental appropriateness rather than age appropriateness, and that age stereotypes and other social and psychological barriers must be eliminated if participation in physical activity is to occur across the life span of each individual.

Declining Physical Activity

REFERENCES

Abrams, B. Advertisers start recognizing cost of insulting elderly. *Wall Street Journal*, March 5, 1981, p. 27.

Albinson, J.G. Attitude measurement in physical education: A review and discussion. In B.S. Rushall (Ed.), *The status of psychomotor learning and sport psychology research*. Halifax, Nova Scotia: Sport Science Associates, 1975.

Atchley, R. Retirement and leisure participation: Continuity or crisis? *The Gerontologist*, 1971, *11*, 13-17.

Atchley, R.C., & Seltzer, M.M. *The sociology of aging: Selected readings*. Belmont, Calif.: Wadsworth, 1976.

Bassey, E.J. Age, inactivity and some physiological responses to exercise. *Gerontology*, 1978, *24*, 66-77.

Bem, S.L. The measurement of psychological androgyny. *Journal of Consulting and Clinical Psychology*, 1974, *42*, 155-162.

Boothby, J., Tungatt, M.F., & Townsend, A.R. Ceasing participation in sports activity: Reported reasons and their implications. *Journal of Leisure Research*, 1981, *13*, 1-14.

Botwinick, J. *Aging and behavior* (2nd ed.). New York: Springer, 1978.

Butler, R.N. Age-ism: Another form of bigotry. *The Gerontologist*, 1969, *9*, 243-246.

Butler, R.N. *Why survive? Being old in America*. New York: Harper & Row, 1975.

Calderone, M.S. Sex and aging. In R. Gross, B. Gross, & S. Seidman (Eds.), *The new old: Struggling for decent aging*. Garden City, N.Y.: Anchor Press, 1978.

Clarke, H.H. (Ed.). National Adult Physical Fitness Survey. *President's Council on Physical Fitness and Sports Newsletter*, 1973, 1-27.

Clarke, H.H. (Ed.). National adult physical fitness survey. *Physical Fitness Research Digest*, 1974, *4*, 1-27.

Comfort, A. Aging: Real and imaginary. In R. Gross, B. Gross, & S. Seidman (Eds.), *The new old: Struggling for decent aging*. Garden City, N.Y.: Anchor Press, 1978.

Conrad, C.C. When you're young at heart. *Aging*, 1976, *258*, 11-13.

Cullen, K.J., & Weeks, P.J. Sporting activities and exercise habits of the 1975 Busselton population. *The Medical Journal of Australia*, 1978, *1*, 69-71.

Cunningham, D.A., Montoye, H.J., Metzner, H.L., & Keller, J.B. Active leisure time activities as related to age among males in a total population. *Journal of Gerontology*, 1968, *23*, 551-556.

Del Rey, P. In support of apologetics for women in sport. In R.W. Christina & D.M. Landers (Eds.), *Psychology of motor behavior and sport—1976*. Champaign, Ill.: Human Kinetics, 1976.

deVries, H.A. *Vigor regained*. Englewood Cliffs, N.J.: Prentice-Hall, 1974.

Ellfeldt, L., & Lowman, C.L. *Exercises for the mature adult*. Springfield, Ill.: Charles C. Thomas, 1973.

Falconer, W.A. (trans.). *Cicero*. Cambridge, Mass.: Harvard University Press, 1964.

Fisher, A.C., Genovese, P.O., Morris, K.J., & Morris, H.H. Perceptions of women in sport. In D.M. Landers & R.W. Christina (Eds.), *Psychology of motor behavior and sport—1977*. Champaign, Ill.: Human Kinetics, 1978.

Gunter, J., & Bratton, R.D. Senior citizens and bowling: A study in motivation. *Review of Sport and Leisure*, 1980, *5*, 70-80.

Harris, D.V. *Involvement in sport: A somatopsychic rationale for physical activity*. Philadelphia: Lea & Febiger, 1973.

Heikkinen, E., & Kayhty, B. Gerontological aspects of physical activity— Motivation of older people in physical training. In R. Harris & L.J. Frankel (Eds.), *Guide to fitness after 50*. New York: Plenum Press, 1977.

Hobart, C.W. Active sports participation among the young, the middle-aged, and the elderly. *International Review of Sport Sociology*, 1975, *10*, 27-44.

Jones, D.C. *The relationship of sex-role orientation to stereotypes held for female athletes in selected sports*. Unpublished doctoral dissertation, West Virginia University, 1979.

Kaplan, M. *Leisure: Lifestyle and lifespan*. Philadelphia: W.B. Saunders, 1979.

Kenyon, G.S. A conceptual model for characterizing physical activity. *Research Quarterly*, 1968, *39*, 96-105. (a)

Kenyon, G.S. Six scales for assessing attitude toward physical activity. *Research Quarterly*, 1968, *39*, 566-574. (b)

Kleiber, D.A., & Kelly, J.R. Leisure, socialization and the life cycle. In S.E. Iso-Ahola (Ed.), *Social psychological perspectives in leisure and recreation*. Springfield, Ill.: Charles C. Thomas, 1980.

Kriete, M.M. *The effects of a static exercise program upon specific joint mobilities in healthy female senior citizens*. Unpublished master's thesis, Springfield College, 1976.

Kuhn, M. New life for the elderly: Liberation from "ageism." In R. Gross, B. Gross, & S. Seidman (Eds.), *The new old: Struggling for decent aging*. Garden City, N.Y.: Anchor Press, 1978.

Levin, J., & Levin, W.C. *Ageism: Prejudice and discrimination against the elderly*. Belmont, Calif.: Wadsworth, 1980.

Lewko, J.H., & Greendorfer, S.L. Family influence and sex differences in children's socialization into sport: A review. In D.M. Landers & R.W. Christina (Eds.), *Psychology of motor behavior and sport—1977*. Champaign, Ill.: Human Kinetics, 1978.

Louis Harris & Associates, Inc. Myths and realities of life for older Americans. In R. Gross, B. Gross, & S. Seidman (Eds.), *The new old: Struggling for decent aging*. Garden City, N.Y.: Anchor Press, 1978.

Ludtke, R.L., O'Leary, T.J., & Wilke, A.S. Activity levels and the fitness account. *Journal of Leisure Research*, 1979, *11*, 207-214.

Maddox, G.L., & Wiley, J. Scope, concepts, and methods in the study of aging. In R.H. Binstock & E. Shanas (Eds.), *Handbook of aging and the social sciences*. New York: Van Nostrand Reinhold, 1976.

Martens, R. Competition: In need of a theory. In D.M. Landers (Ed.), *Social problems in athletics*. Urbana: University of Illinois Press, 1976.

McPherson, B.D. Aging and involvement in physical activity: A sociological perspective. In F. Landry & W. Orban (Eds.), *Physical activity and human wellbeing*. Miami, Fla.: Symposia Specialists, 1978.

McPherson, B.D., & Kozlik, C.A. Canadian leisure patterns by age: Disengagement, continuity, or ageism? In V.W. Marshall (Ed.), *Aging in Canada: Social perspectives*. Pickering, Ontario: Fitzhenry & Whiteside, 1980.

McTavish, D.G. Perceptions of old people. A review of research methodologies and findings. *The Gerontologist*, 1971, *11*, 90–108.

Montoye, H.J. *Physical activity and health: An epidemiologic study of an entire community*. Englewood Cliffs, N.J.: Prentice-Hall, 1975.

Neugarten, B.L. Acting one's age: New rules for old. *Psychology Today*, 1980, *14*, 66–80.

Neugarten, B.L., & Datan, N. Sociological perspectives on the life cycle. In P.B. Baltes & K.W. Schaie (Eds.), *Life-span developmental psychology: Personality and socialization*. New York: Academic Press, 1973.

Neugarten, B.L., & Hagestad, G.O. Age and the life course. In R.H. Binstock & E. Shanas (Eds.) *Handbook of aging and the social sciences*. New York: Van Nostrand Reinhold, 1976.

Nielsen, A.B. *Physical activity patterns of senior citizens*. Unpublished master's thesis, University of Alberta, 1974.

Ostrow, A.C. *Validation of a conceptual model characterizing attitudes of the elderly toward lifetime sports: A preliminary report*. Paper presented at the Midwest American Alliance for Health, Physical Education, and Recreation Convention, Madison, Wis., 1979.

Ostrow, A.C. Physical activity as it relates to the health of the aged. In N. Datan & N. Lohmann (Eds.), *Transitions of aging*. New York: Academic Press, 1980.

Ostrow, A.C. Age role stereotyping: Implications for physical activity participation. In G. Rowles & R. Ohta (Eds.), *Aging and milieu: Environmental perspectives on growing old*. New York: Academic Press, 1983.

Ostrow, A.C., Jones, D.C., & Spiker, D.D. Age role expectations and sex role expectations for selected sport activities. *Research Quarterly for Exercise and Sport*, 1981, *52*, 216–227.

Ostrow, A.C., & Spiker, D.D. *The stereotyping of sport participation based on age role and sex role appropriateness*. Paper presented at the North American Society for the Psychology of Sport and Physical Activity annual convention, Monterey, Calif., 1981.

Palmore, E.B. The effects of aging on activities and attitudes. *The Gerontologist*, 1968, *8*, 263.

Palmore, E.B. Predictors of successful aging. *The Gerontologist*, 1979, *19*, 427–431.

Pasini, G. Sport in old age. *Journal of Sports Medicine and Physical Fitness*, 1975, *15*, 170–171.

Pullias, E.V. Problems of aging: Psychological principles. *Journal of Physical Education and Recreation*, 1977, *48*, 33–35.

Riley, M.W. Social gerontology and the age stratification of society. *The Gerontologist*, 1971, *11*, 79–87.

Riley, M.W. Age strata in social systems. In R.H. Binstock & E. Shanas (Eds.), *Handbook of aging and the social sciences*. New York: Van Nostrand Reinhold, 1976.

Riley, M.W., & Waring, J. Most of the problems of aging are not biological, but social. In R. Gross, B. Gross, & S. Seidman (Eds.), *The new old: Struggling for decent aging.* Garden City, N.Y.: Anchor Press, 1978.

Scanlan, T.K. Social evaluation: A key developmental element in the competitive process. In R.A. Magill, M.J. Ash, & F.L. Smoll (Eds.), *Children in sport: A contemporary anthology.* Champaign, Ill.: Human Kinetics, 1978.

Shephard, R.J., & Sidney, K.H. Exercise and aging. In R. Hutton (Ed.), *Exercise and sport science reviews* (Vol. 7). Philadelphia: Franklin Institute Press, 1979.

Sidney, K.H., & Shephard, R.J. Attitudes toward health and physical activity in the elderly. Effects of a physical training program. *Medicine and Science in Sports,* 1976, *8,* 246-252.

Sidney, K.H., & Shephard, R.J. Activity patterns of elderly men and women. *Journal of Gerontology,* 1977, *32,* 25-32.

Smith, E.L., & Serfass, R.C. (Eds.). *Exercise and aging.* Hillside, N.J.: Enslow, 1981.

Snyder, E.E. *A reflection on commitment and patterns of disengagement from recreational physical activity.* Paper presented at the North American Society for the Sociology of Sport convention, Denver, 1980.

Swanson, M.B. *Physical activity attitudes of senior citizens.* Unpublished master's thesis, University of Montana, 1976.

Teague, M.L. Aging and leisure: A social psychological perspective. In S.E. Iso-Ahola (Ed.), *Social psychological perspectives on leisure and recreation.* Springfield, Ill.: Charles C. Thomas, 1980.

Trippatt, F. Looking askance at ageism. *Time,* March 24, 1980, p. 88.

Trowbridge, B.M. *The effect of a selected exercise program on the attitudes of elderly men toward exercise and physical activity.* Unpublished doctoral dissertation, University of Oregon, 1978.

Winer, F. The elderly jock and how he got that way. In J.H. Goldstein (Ed.), *Sports, games, and play: Social and psychological viewpoints.* Hillsdale, N.J.: Lawrence Erlbaum, 1979.

6

Physical Activity Programs for the Older Adult

This chapter deals with the development of physical activity programs for the older adult. In the first part of this chapter, I review selected programs that now exist in the United States. This review is not meant to be all-encompassing;* rather, these programs were selected because they illustrate the diversity of physical activities available to the older adult. I then outline a set of program principles and concomitant recommendations to guide the formulation of programs of physical activity for the older adult. My goal is to attempt to synthesize and apply some of the information presented previously in this book so that program recommendations are based on sound theoretical and empirical evidence rather than on armchair philosophizing. I conclude this chapter with a set of guidelines for training future leaders in the field of physical activity and aging.

EXISTING PROGRAMS

Project Preventicare

Late in 1970, with financial assistance from the West Virginia State Commission on Aging, Lawrence Frankel and his colleagues were charged with developing a physical fitness program for the elderly. A pilot study of 15 subjects, who ranged in age from 60 to 80 years, was initiated. Based on these initial results, Project Preventicare was spawned (Frankel, 1977).

Project Preventicare represents a low-level series of mobility exercises that can be adapted to both ambulatory older individuals and those more debilitated in movement. The program is described in great depth in a book entitled *Be Alive as Long as You Live* (Frankel & Richard, 1977). Activities are designed for those over 60 years of age. Most of the program activities appear to be targeted toward flexibility and muscular strength changes, although there are some cardiorespiratory endurance activities.

*See the appendix for a reference list of physical activity programs and related training resources for the older adult prepared for the National Clearinghouse on Aging.

139

Interval training is included, but the authors caution that the heart rate should not exceed 100–120 beats/minute; subjects are encouraged and instructed on how to self-monitor their heart rates. All participants in the program have their heart rate and blood pressure recorded every 2 weeks. Music is used to enhance both mood and tolerance while exercising. Physician approval is a prerequisite for participation in the program. The authors say that, although there may be some risk in activity, there is more risk in inactivity.

The Preventicare program was initially designed to reach older people in outlying communities, federally built housing complexes, and the institutionalized elderly within the state of West Virginia (Frankel, 1977). It was geared particularly to a clientele, who, for the most part, were not fortunate enough to have participated in sport, physical education, or recreation during their lifetimes. Thousands of individuals have participated in the program, and there is growing, worldwide interest (Frankel & Richard, 1977).

The Oaknoll Exercise Society

The Oaknoll Exercise Society (TOES) program, described by Leslie and McClure (1975) in their booklet *Exercises for the Elderly*, comprises a series of low-stress exercises designed to "tone up muscles, improve joint articulation, promote relaxation, help rid people of constipation, and give a sense of well-being" (p. 1). Originally formed in response to the physical activity needs of members of the Oaknoll Retirement Residence in Iowa City, Iowa, the program, through a Title III grant under the Older American's Act, has expanded to include a seven-county area around Iowa City. In addition, TOES became part of an educational television network series.

Activities have been conducted, for the most part, indoors. The socializing benefits of participation are emphasized. Participation in group programs requires physician approval. Bands, wands, surgical tubing, boxes, and plastic bottles are examples of equipment that can be adapted for use in the exercise program. Music is encouraged while exercising. Exercise leaders are recommended when the program is conducted in a group setting.

Participants are told to try to exercise at least two to three times a week for approximately 30–40 minutes each session. Guidelines are provided for selecting appropriate exercises based on the entry fitness level and interest of the individual. Participants are encouraged to include a variety of exercises in their repertoire to ensure that all body parts are active. Exercises in the program are classified by body part into 1 of 14 categories, and participants are instructed to sample from each category. They are also encouraged to create their own exercises. The authors suggest that evaluations of the program should be made periodically by all those involved.

Adults' Health and Developmental Program

The Adults' Health and Developmental Program (AHDP), developed and directed by Dan Leviton, is an "interdisciplinary, intergenerational approach to health maintenance and improvement" (Leviton, 1977, p. 33). It incorporates a gamut of physical activities and is located at the University of Maryland, College Park. Inexpensive to operate and simple in design, it provides health-related services to older adults and also serves as a training ground for students interested in gerontological health and research. Turnover for students (staff) and older adult members is low. The program is viewed as providing preventive, interventive, and postventive (or rehabilitative) health care (Leviton, 1974, 1977).

The ADHP "aims to improve the physical basis of personality through social interaction in an environment of fun and joy" (Leviton, 1977, p. 34). For example, it seeks to improve the self-concept of the older adult through the provision of physical activities that are individually prescribed to enhance his/her body image. The emphasis is on individually prescribed activity and between 45 and 60 students from every discipline volunteer to help (and learn) during the Saturday morning sessions. Older adults are encouraged to acquire new motor skills or relearn old ones. Health discussions are also held, providing further opportunities for young and old to share their concerns and perspectives on such issues as nutrition, consumer education, and human sexuality. Between 45 and 60 older adults participate in the program each semester. A film entitled "Smiles: The Adults' Health and Developmental Program" nicely illustrates the program and is available for purchase from the University of Maryland.

NAHD-PCPFS Exercises

A series of 23 exercises for older adults, emphasizing flexibility, balance, and muscular strength, have been prepared by the National Association for Human Development (NAHD) and the President's Council for Physical Fitness and Sports (PCPFS). These exercises have frequently been adopted in programs of physical activity for the older adult (e.g. Jable & Cheesman, 1978) and in research projects (e.g., Parks, 1979). The exercise program is described in a booklet entitled *The Fitness Challenge... in the Later Years* (1975) prepared by the PCPFS and the Administration on Aging.

The booklet begins with a quote from an eminent physician: "Most of us don't wear out, we rust out" (p. i). The values of remaining physically fit as we grow older are extolled, and fitness programming principles, such as the need for progressive, systematic exercise and the importance of properly "warming up," are reviewed. The exercises are graded according to the degree of difficulty or the amount of stress involved. Three program levels are established: the Red (easiest) program, the White program, and the Blue (most difficult) program. Individuals self-

141

select their appropriate program entry levels based on physician advice and a series of self-administered walk-jog tests. Advice is given on setting program goals and self-monitoring participation in the exercise regimen. Individuals are encouraged to add other physical activities to their exercise schedule.

Fitness Trail

Recognizing that traditional aerobic training programs involve a high rate of attrition among older adults (because of loss of interest, recurrence of medical problems, and other factors), the recreation coordinator of Waukesha, Wisconsin, and researchers at the University of Wisconsin developed a Fitness Trail program that was conveniently set up in a nearby county park (Morse & Smith, 1981). Based on a medical examination and ECG and submaximal treadmill tests, older adults are placed in small groups of four or five individuals. Each group is assigned a fitness trail of appropriate difficulty to walk in the park. Initially, each trail is subdivided into quarter-mile lengths, with strength and flexibility exercise stations located at rest intervals. All groups attempt to complete the entire exercise circuit at the same time, thus ensuring, because the trails vary in fitness demands, differential exercise bouts among the established groups.

During the program, blood pressures at rest are assessed weekly, and participants are asked to self-monitor their heart rates during the exercise circuit. Sessions are 1 hour each and are held three times a week. The program convenes early in the morning during the summer to avoid the problems associated with hyperthermia in the elderly. Spouses and close friends are urged to attend to improve attendance and minimize attrition. Furthermore, the park setting provides a convenient and aesthetically pleasing environment in which to exercise.

Discussion

This brief review of some available physical activity and exercise programs is not meant to be all-inclusive; rather, the intent is to illustrate the diversity of programs that have been initiated across the country. There have been other physical activity programs for the older adult reported in the literature. For example, Garnet (1982) discusses her Geriatric Body Dynamics program, a holistic movement therapy program for motorically impaired older adults, in her book, *Movement Is Life.* Corbin (1981) and Hattlestad (1979) review ongoing exercise prescription programs for the older adult. There are also competitive programs, such as the Senior Olympics, for the more skilled older athlete (Kamm, 1979).

For the most part, current physical activity programs for the older adult appear to be exercise prescription programs with a primary focus on developing and maintaining physical fitness. I have used the words "appear to be" very carefully, because often it is difficult to interpret what the intended purposes of these programs really are. Program objectives and criteria for meeting these objectives are noticeably absent from many program descriptions. Although many of the activities employed with older adults appear to have some relationship to developing physical fitness, it is often unclear as to what specific components of fitness (e.g., muscular strength, flexibility) each activity is expected to enhance. It is almost as if the program leader hopes that a potpourri of physical activities will inevitably contribute to the fitness welfare (or at least the social welfare) of the older adult. In other words, the philosophy seems to be that something is better than nothing. However, if we are to develop valid, worthwhile programs of exercise, and more importantly, if we are to gain the confidence and interest of older members of our society in exercise, then exercise prescription must be based on carefully documented scientific evidence. Certainly, as Chapter 4 showed, fitness changes are contingent upon the use of appropriately designed physical activities that are specifically targeted toward desired physical fitness outcomes. Most programs lack adequate scientific documentation as to their effectiveness.

It is disappointing to note how few physical activities programs emphasize motor skill acquisition and development among the elderly. Some program leaders would vehemently argue that their programs are designed to teach the older adult new motor skills. However, the developmental perspective of some activity programs suggests that the aging process inevitably brings us back to performing childhood motor skills. For example, in one program (to remain anonymous) nursing home residents "popped" nerf balls and small yarn balls through a parachute, played tug-of-war, rolled beach balls at each other, tossed large rings at upturned chairs, and then had cookies and lemonade. While I am sure these activities are well intended and thought to promote fun and social interaction, we must never forget that older adults have needs that are different from those of young children. Professionals are doing our older generation a disservice if they think that "fun and games" is the answer to the older adult's motor development and enrichment.

Most programs suffer from a lack of adequate information on how to best meet the physical activity needs of the older adult. For example, it is now recognized, particularly as a result of the extensive factor analytic research investigations of Fleishman (1964, 1966, 1967, 1972) and Rarick and his colleagues (Rarick & Dobbins, 1975; Rarick, Dobbins, & Broadhead, 1976; Rarick & McQuillan, 1977), that a number of common and specific psychomotor abilities underlie the execution of a wide range of physical proficiency skills among children and young adults. It is generally assumed that, although these psychomotor abilities become more differentiated, they are not likely to change once adulthood is reached (Fleishman, 1966; Singer, 1975). It is conceivable, however, that age-related declines in motor *skill* are symptomatic of corresponding age-related declines in psychomotor *ability*. In other words, observed motor performance declines as a function of age may be due, in part, to changes in the underlying contributions of balance, coordination, and other abilities to specific motor performances as we grow older. Surprisingly, there have been no systematic efforts to extend the research of Fleishman and Rarick across the life cycle to determine if, in fact, the factor structure of psychomotor abilities does remain stable.

There have been some attempts (e.g., Shivers & Fait, 1980) to categorize sport activities into speed sports, body control sports, and other types, but at this point these categories lack adequate scientific verification. We really do not know what kinds of abilities can most readily be improved in older persons, nor the conditions and tasks most likely to facilitate these changes.

Within recent years, there has been a concerted effort by the American Alliance for Health, Physical Education, Recreation, and Dance (AAHPERD) to accelerate activities that serve the elderly in this country ("Alliance programs," 1979). These activities have included

1. an expanded information clearinghouse to cover the full range of health, fitness, and leisure service programs for older adults
2. "News Kit on Programs for Aging," which appears twice a year as part of the newsletter *Update*
3. the development of a film entitled "Health, Fitness and Leisure for a Quality Life" to stimulate community health and fitness programs
4. the sponsorship of a nationwide series of workshops on physical activity and the older adult
5. cooperative endeavors with other agencies and organizations concerned with health, fitness, and leisure services for older adults

Linkages between the AAHPERD Committee on Aging and the AAHPERD Research Consortium, and between other research-oriented organizations such as the North American Society for the Psychology of Sport and Physical Activity (NASPSPA), can ensure that a concomitant research base evolves to support emerging programs of physical activity for the older adult. Without this network, program specialists risk being chastised by the scientific community for providing unsafe and unsubstantiated activity delivery systems, and "turning off" future generations of older adults from remaining physically active.

PRINCIPLES AND RECOMMENDATIONS

What characteristics of the older adult must be considered when discussing the programming of physical activity? Butler (1975), in his Pulitzer-Prize-winning book, *Why Survive? Being Old in America,* presented a realistic portrayal of our older clientele. He pointed out that they are as diverse as people in other periods of life, but that old age is characterized by complex and rapidly occurring changes that can have overwhelming effects. Yet, whether these changes are a result of disease, life experience, or socioeconomic and other factors, most older adults learn to live with these changes through various coping strategies. He also indicated:

Older people are apt to be reflective rather than impulsive. Having experienced a great deal and having been "burned often," they think before acting. Under suitable circumstances, the present remains very much alive and exciting to them; but they also turn to a review of their past, searching for purpose, reconciliation of relationships and resolution of conflicts and regrets. They may become self-centered or altruistic, angry or contrite, triumphant or depressed.

Those old people who are optimistic and resourceful may at the same time be painfully aware of the brevity of life and its tragedies. Optimism is tempered by a more balanced view of the joys and sadnesses of life. The old continue to learn and change in response to their experiences and to human relationships. They are not often overwhelmed by new ideas for they recognize how few of them there are. Many are employable, productive and creative. Many wish to leave their mark through sponsoring the young as well as through ideas and institutions. (Butler, 1975, p. 408)

These characteristics of being old in America should be kept in mind as I review a number of important principles and recommendations germane to programming physical activity for the older adult. It should be obvious to the reader that programming physical activity for the older adult requires more care and thought than for any other age group (Morse & Smith, 1981).

Principle 1. Older adults, for the most part, bring to a physical activities program a history rich in physical inactivity.

A small number of older adults have religiously adhered to a lifetime of vigorous physical activity, and an even smaller number continue to compete in sanctioned athletic events. Most older adults, however, gradually disengaged from physical activity as they grew older. Morse and Smith (1981) suggested that when prescribing physical activity and, in particular, when determining exercise intensity we should consider

145

the following categories: (a) the "old" old, those individuals over 75 years of age who may need the support environment of a nursing home; (b) the "young" old, those individuals approximately 60–75 years of age who reside in their own homes and who are still able to maintain active lifestyles; and (c) the athletic old, those rare individuals who have maintained a high level of physical fitness and who are still competitively active in sport. These categorizations certainly alert physical activity leaders to the potential diversity of older adult clientele.

Recommendation 1. The older adult should be medically screened prior to participation in a physical activities program.

Guidelines developed by the AAHPERD Committee on Aging make clear the potential risks of the sudden, unregulated, and injudicious use of exercise in the elderly. The committee recommends that for programs involving vigorous exercise the preliminary medical evaluation should ensure that the older adult can participate without any undue risk to the cardiovascular and other bodily systems. For participation in physical activity programs involving low-intensity exercise (i.e., exercises that do not exceed the level of intensity encountered in normal daily activities), the older adult should at least have physician approval.

A preliminary stress test is particularly important prior to older adult participation in a physical activities program having a high aerobic component. This test not only identifies high-risk subjects, but also permits an initial functional estimate for activity prescription. Montoye (1975) outlined a number of criteria that mandated a stress test and/or led to activity exclusion. These criteria included a history of myocardial infarction, angina pectoris, or congestive heart failure; insulin therapy; vasodilating drug medication; and orthopedic disabilities. Morse and Smith (1981) provided an excellent overview of the concerns and limitations of various stress tests (such as treadmill testing, bicycling testing, and step testing) when used with older adults. They indicated that reduced aerobic capacity, mobility, and neuromuscular function necessitated a modified testing method among older adults.

Physician evaluation of the individual's medical history, the participant's self-evaluation, and the results of a stress test are all important ingredients of a preliminary screening. As deVries (1976) has noted, using only one of these screening tools may provide an inadequate prediction of the older adult's response to vigorous physical activity.

Recommendation 2. Physical activity must be progressive and adapted to each individual's tolerance level.

Differing fitness entry levels and previous activity experiences mandate that professionals do *not* homogenize older adult physical activity programs. However, the optimum exercise regimen for the improvement

146

of physical fitness has yet to be defined, even among younger subjects (Shephard & Sidney, 1979). Similarly, at this point we have little information on how motor skills can be fractionated sequentially so that optimal performance is achieved.

The American College of Sports Medicine (ACSM, 1978) has issued a position statement on the recommended quantity and quality of exercise for developing and maintaining fitness in healthy adults. They have also published excellent guidelines for exercise testing and training adults (ACSM, 1975). This organization notes that with respect to developing and maintaining cardiorespiratory fitness and body composition, exercise prescription should be based upon the frequency, intensity, and duration of training, the mode of activity, and initial fitness levels. Frequency of exercise is recommended at 3-5 days/week, and the minimal threshold for improvement in $\dot{V}O_2\,_{max}$ is approximately 60 percent of the maximum heart rate reserve. This threshold may be as low as 110-120 beats/minute for older persons, particularly those who have been inactive. Exercise must be maintained on a regular basis to avoid reductions in working capacity. The impact of age and fitness level on resulting detraining effects is unclear at this point. However, age, in itself, does not appear to be a deterrent to endurance training. Older adults may need longer periods of time to adapt to training.

There is little, if any, information available on optimum training regimens for older adults on other fitness parameters such as muscular strength and flexibility. Furthermore, there is a lack of data on what variables facilitate "new" skill acquisition and the relearning of "old" skills among older adults. The impact of previous training on subsequent skill acquisition is unclear. Valid diagnostic tools to assess motor development adequately in the elderly are nonexistent. Thus, the program leader must rely heavily on intuition and experience when developing a sequentially graded set of motor activities that lead to progressive skill attainment among older adults.

Recommendation 3. The older adult's participation in physical activity must be carefully monitored.

The risks attendant with physical activity, particularly vigorous physical activity, are greater among the elderly. Thus, the AAHPERD Committee on Aging recommends that each person's response to exercise be carefully monitored periodically for signs of undue stress (such as nausea, pain, high heart rate, and/or dyspnea). Older adults can and should be taught to monitor their own heart rates and to recognize indicators of stress. There are a number of digital, commercial devices that can be used conveniently by the older adult to monitor heart rate levels during exercise. This self-monitoring process may also motivate the older adult to sustain or gradually increase workload rates.

Exercise programs must be adequately supervised by personnel who are trained in cardiopulmonary resuscitation (CPR) techniques. Furthermore, as the AAHPERD Committee on Aging notes, activity leaders must have well-defined emergency plans to follow in the event of cardiac arrest or other accidents. There is an obvious employment opportunity here for athletic trainers who have an interest in gerontology. Their availability during activity would help to minimize the risks of injury, strains, and sprains, which affect mobility more adversely with advancing age.

Principle 2. Older adults evidence greater variability on most parameters related to physical activity participation.

A consistent theme that emerged from Chapter 3 was that with increasing age, individuals exhibited greater heterogeneity in RT, movement speed, physical fitness, and other parameters related to physical activity. To homogenize physical activity programs and to slot older adults into a common set of activities as if they were all alike would be a terrible injustice to them and would surely decrease their enthusiasm for remaining physically active.

Recommendation 4. Physical activity programs for the older adult should be based on an individually prescribed instructional (IPI) system.

The IPI system is an instructional method of individualizing program components to ensure the optimal development of each program participant, and it has received much attention as a logical solution to the mainstreaming of handicapped children within a physical education classroom environment (Auxter, 1971; Bundschuh & Wiegand, 1975; Rarick & McQuillan, 1977; Wiegand, 1977). By law, each handicapped child must have a written individual educational program (IEP) including, among other things, relevant assessment data, long-term goals, short-term instructional objectives, and evaluative criteria. The IPI system would seem to be a logical solution to individualizing physical activity programs for the older adult. Unfortunately, most programs of physical activity reviewed in this chapter have adopted a group approach to meeting the activity needs of the older adult. Programming centers around group games, group-led exercises, and group sport participation. This approach leaves little room for enriching the motor development of older adults whose motor abilities may have become more diverse with advancing age.

An effective IPI system to enhance the motor development of the older adult must be based on a sound and empirically derived conceptual model representative of the broad range of motor abilities of older adults. In that hierarchically sequenced activity programs are the basis of any IPI system, these activity programs must be representative of these motor abilities and must contain valid, hierarchically sequenced behavioral objectives. Furthermore, these objectives must lead to a valid and reliable means of assessing whether the older adult is progressing through the activity sequence.

I am not aware of any methodological research designed to develop and examine the effectiveness of an IPI system within an older adult physical activity program. Such an endeavor is needed to improve the credibility of these programs and to meet the diverse needs of each participant.

Recommendation 5. Assignments to physical activities must be based on developmental readiness rather than on age alone.

The assignment of individuals (including older adults) to program categories has frequently been made on the basis of chronological age rather than developmental appropriateness. Of course, chronological age offers a convenient and quick means of expediting activity assignment. However, individual systems age at different rates, and there are many potential indices of aging other than chronological age. If programming is to respond adequately to variations in the aging process, program specialists must be more creative in the manner by which they diagnose the "aged" person.

Maturation matching may be one solution to this problem. Skeletal age is the most reliable method for matching on the basis of physical maturity, particularly among the young, but it poses problems of cost and the additional health hazard of radiation exposure. One classification scheme described by Martens (1978), called the Selection Classification Age Maturity Program (SCAM), has been successfully used in the New York State public school sports program. Young children entering the program are matched on the basis of physical fitness, skills, and physical maturity. This system has been successful in reducing injury. There is no reason why this classification approach cannot be adapted to individuals at the other end of the life cycle. Of course, as Martens pointed out, one would still need to determine the acceptable ranges in maturity for grouping people together in sport and for permitting individuals to self-select certain physical activities.

Another approach to classifying older adults developmentally might be based on the determination of each individual's *motoric age*. Motoric age might best be defined as the psychomotor functional capacity of the individual at a given point in the life cycle. Procedures used by Borkan and Norris (1980) in their assessment of biological age might also be extrapolated to determine one's motoric age. Age-sensitive variables in a motoric test battery could be employed in a regression analysis. The resulting residual scores would be standardized, allowing the conversion

149

of a number of age-related variables (in the test battery) to motoric age scores. These motoric age scores would be averaged across individuals, resulting in a motoric age index for each individual. Using this approach, it is possible to find that two individuals who differ in chronological age are quite similar with respect to motoric age.

I think we need to be more creative in how we approach the question of developmental readiness, particularly among older adults. A heavy reliance on chronological age as a criterion for physical activity assignment may have resulted in participant mismatching and frustrations on the part of many older adults.

Recommendation 6. Physical activity choices must be based on facts rather than on myths.

An important corollary to Recommendation 5 is the need to select rationally physical activities that address the developmental needs of each older adult. It would be a mistake to state that all older adults should avoid vigorous aerobic activity, weight training, or cross-country skiing. Previous experience, fitness history, and interest should also be determinants of participation. To reiterate, however, it is very difficult to prescribe an appropriate diet of physical activity for elderly people when the scientific evidence regarding the capacities and needs of older age groups is so sparse.

Selection of an appropriate mode of activity is particularly important with respect to older adults. Greater proneness to the potential debilitating effects of injury, and decrements in fitness, sensory processes, and motor performance, mandate that program leaders exercise wisdom in the assignment of people to activities.

The ACSM (1978) stated that "any activity that uses large muscle groups, that can be maintained continuously, and is rhythmical and aerobic in nature" (p. vii), such as running-jogging, swimming, bicycling, and rowing, can enhance and maintain cardiorespiratory fitness. It is also true, however, that endurance activities requiring running and jumping increase the risk of orthopedic injuries and should probably be avoided among older adults who have been physically inactive. As Morse and Smith (1981) advised, walking-hiking, swimming, and aerobic dancing may be more appropriate activities for most older adults. The reader might want to review carefully Piscopo's (1979) suggestions regarding the contraindications and indications of appropriate physical activity for the older adult.

As I noted in Chapter 3, older adults have achievement needs that can be expressed through physical activity. It is wrong, therefore, to suggest that competition should be avoided among *all* older adults. I think there has been an overestimation of the impact of aging when prescribing physical activities for the older adult. Future generations of elderly who, it is hoped, have remained physically active during their life course may be placed on a less restricted diet of physical activity.

Principle 3. Whether due to age, inactivity, and/or disease, most older adults exhibit marked decrements on most parameters related to physical activity participation.

In planning programs of physical activity, professionals must not overlook the fact that older adults, on the average, are less ambulatory than younger populations. There are age-related declines in most sensory systems, in central nervous system processing, and in resulting RT and movement speed responses. Regardless of the causes of these declines, of central importance to programming is the manner by which these decrements are addressed within a learning environment that still allows for the optimal development of physical activity and fitness-related skills.

Recommendation 7. The program leader must provide an effective delivery system for the learning and maintenance of motor skills.

Declines in visual acuity accelerate after 50 years of age; older people need greater levels of illumination and cannot see as well in the dark. Thus, the physical activity setting should be well lighted, particularly if classes are held in the evening. Written instructions and signs should contain large lettering. The program leader should ensure that those participants afflicted with presbyopia are wearing proper eyeglasses.

Hearing impairments are more common than visual impairments after 65 years of age. Older people have greater difficulty understanding speech, particularly in noisy environments. Thus, activities which require whisper signals (such as relays) and a lot of verbal directions should be avoided (Piscopo, 1979). The pace of instructions should be slower, allowing adequate time for central processing. More repetition of verbal directions may be required (Shivers & Fait, 1980).

The program leader should rely more heavily on nonverbal communication. Persons who are hearing impaired may want to see the lips of the program leader in order to "read" them. It may be necessary to speak very close to the ear, and one ear may be the "good ear." Furthermore, touch and tactile communication may increase the responsiveness of the older person to activity (Butler & Lewis, 1977). Manual guidance should be used to help the older person "feel" the desired movement.

Listening is an important skill for program leaders to develop and practice. Many older people have a great deal to talk about and frequently reminisce (Butler & Lewis, 1977). Social interaction between participants should be encouraged. The program leader should let the older person verbalize his/her feelings about the activity. Exaggerated fears of activity should be resolved. Under the direction of a professionally trained activities (or sport) counselor, systematic strategies can be developed to help the individual and group deal with feelings of anxiety and apprehension, and the activity can be structured to maximize emotional relaxation. These procedures may serve to increase participant attentiveness and decrease cautiousness, two behaviors commonly confused with hearing impairment and slowness of movement among the elderly.

The program leader should be alert to reductions in proprioceptive sensitivity which affect the older person's sense of position and balance. Activities demanding precise static body balance movements, such as standing on one foot with eyes closed, should be avoided. Balance beam activities, if safely structured, may enhance balance skills (Piscopo, 1979). The program leader should remove obstacles and structure the learning environment to reduce the dangers of falls and injury among the elderly.

Recommendation 8. Counseling skills are an important adjunct to the physical activity program environment.

The decline in motor skills that most older people evidence may precipitate a number of negative emotional responses to the learning environment. Physical activities, particularly those that are not self-paced, that demand rapid decisions and changes in direction, or that are novel or competitive in nature may be particularly stressful to the older adult. This, in turn, may lead to frequent errors, extreme caution, avoidance behaviors, and eventual withdrawal from the program.

Older adults often have low physical self-esteem, and they may underestimate their own abilities to perform. Fear of injury sometimes leads to exaggerated perceptions of risk. Furthermore, older people who have had a history of competing successfully in sport may be particularly vulnerable to the ravages of aging. Some of these individuals may not have readjusted their competitive goals in line with their declining abilities. Encouraging them to compete, without adequate planning and counseling, may be extremely detrimental to their self-perception and welfare.

Since many leaders of older adult physical activity programs lack adequate training in psychology and related areas, support personnel may be needed. An activities counselor, with a strong background in counseling and psychology, can assist the program leader in selecting and sequencing physical activities that are least stressful for the program participant. The counselor can also instruct participants in deep-breathing exercises, progressive relaxation, and other somatic anxiety reduction techniques. Cognitive therapies such as thought stopping and cognitive restructuring can be used to help the participant reconcile irrational fears of injury or failure during activity.

In short, a successful physical activities program adopts a holistic approach to promoting physical activity. There must be a recognition that the prescription of physical activity requires systematic attention to both the head and the body.

Principle 4. Older adults generally exhibit less motivation than younger people toward sustaining participation in physical activity.

Human aging has traditionally been viewed as a period of decline. This perspective has been reinforced by the ubiquitous decline in motor skill participation and performance with advancing age. Attitudinal and social expectancies dictate less physically active life-styles as we grow older. It is no wonder then that a major task facing the program specialist is how to motivate older adults to participate and sustain participation in physical activity.

Recommendation 9. Older adults should be encouraged to set realistic performance goals.

An important source of participant motivation is the successful attainment of individually prescribed goals. An emerging body of literature on goal-setting behavior (e.g., Ostrow, 1976) emphasizes that those individuals who respond successfully to physical activity set realistic, attainable performance goals that are achieved gradually. Conversely, those individuals who sharply underestimate or overestimate their performance abilities, and who set unrealistic goals, typically experience frustration and failure. These individuals sometimes exhibit rigid expectations and refuse to adjust their goals in response to success or failure.

The program leader should help each participant formulate a set of reasonable goals at the outset of the program. Lundegren (1980) concluded that adults are motivated to continue participation in physical activity for reasons related to health and fitness, social contacts, achievement of well-being, improvement of self-image, fun and enjoyment, and feedback on achievement. The relative importance of each of these motives to participation should be identified. Too often, specialists have made the assumption that participant motives are compatible with the goals of the program leader. An individually prescribed sequence of activity, relevant to the needs of each participant, should be developed based on a mutual evaluation of the participant's previous activity history, current fitness and skill levels, and future aspirations. Criteria for attaining a given level of physical fitness or skill development within a reasonable time frame should be established. Process-oriented goals, such as effort, form, or strategy, should also be evaluated (Feltz & Weiss, 1982).

Successful achievement of goals should lead to gradual increments in expectations. The effects of goal nonattainment on loss of self-esteem should be minimized. Group discussions among peers can facilitate feedback on the feasibility of individual goals. The program leader must reinforce the notion that failing is a healthful sign of growing and determine if future goals need to be lower. Discrepancies between program leader and participant goals should be openly discussed.

The procedure outlined here may help sustain the participant's interest in the program. The participant's self-efficacy (e.g., Feltz & Weiss, 1982) is enhanced through self-directed attention to performance outcomes. Estimates of self-worth are enhanced through open discussions of success and failure experiences. Social evaluation among peers is channeled into positive goal adjustments within an individualized program setting. The goal-setting process, in itself, becomes a healthful and important source of self-motivation.

Recommendation 10. Multifaceted strategies must be adopted to sustain older adult interest in physical activity.

In Chapter 4, I reviewed a number of research studies purportedly designed to enhance the mental health of the older adult through physical activity participation. A major drawback to many of these studies was that there were no planned, systematic strategies to impart favorable mental health outcomes. It is not surprising, therefore, that several of these projects suffered from subject attrition. Physical activity, in itself, cannot sustain participant interest or contribute to impressive mental health gains. The program environment must be structured to elicit these outcomes.

A number of program techniques have been employed to sustain older adult interest in physical activity. For example, music is frequently used to accompany exercise regimens. Whitehouse (1977) noted the importance of latitude, self-selection, and novelty in contributing to the older adult's sense of mastery and personal choice. He also emphasized the importance of providing participants with frequent information on performance improvements. The program leader should also encourage participant feedback prior to each session.

Franklin (1978) observed that most exercise programs are short on education. People are told they must exercise, but little information is provided on why or how they should exercise. Participants need information on clothing, nutrition, sleep, and the contraindications of exercise. Franklin proposed the use of bulletin boards, minilectures, fitness newsletters, and educational meetings as integral to the program package. To motivate participants, he recommended that spouses or close friends become involved in the program to provide mutual support, that workouts be held with regularity, and that participants self-monitor their gains through progress charts.

One of the strengths of the Fitness Trail program I reported on earlier was its convenient and aesthetically pleasing location. There are advantages in locating physical activity programs in senior centers or other sites adjacent to ongoing social activities. When facilities are not conveniently located, transportation must be provided for the older adult.

These program suggestions highlight the importance of adequate planning to maximize interest among older adults in participating in physical activity. Many other strategies are possible.

Principle 5. Older adults are adults first and old second.
It should never be forgotten that older adults are adults first and old second. Although they may exhibit diminished motor skills and be incapacitated by the ravages of disease and inactivity, they are still mature individuals witnessing the last stages of their life cycle. Their needs are adult needs, their reflections are adult reflections, and their hopes and aspirations represent the wisdom of their time. We must never degrade their worth through our own prejudices and stereotypes of aging.

Older adults seek acceptance in themselves. They abhor the condescending and patronizing behaviors that so often characterize others in their social environment. Treasure their self-respect. Seek out the wisdom of their years. Do not promise physical activity as the new fountain of youth; for it is not youth, but happiness in old age, that may be most cherished by the older adult.

TRAINING PHYSICAL ACTIVITY LEADERS

Several years ago, I received a letter from a colleague at a university in Colorado who shared his excitement about establishing a physical activities program at a local nursing home. The program was started by a graduate student who was doing an internship project. The results were so fantastic that the director of the home requested additional students. The residents "felt more cheerful, happier and appeared in better spirits as a result of the program." Unfortunately, there was a lack of university support, and the program was discontinued pending extramural funding. My colleague wrote that the residents used to look for the students an hour before they arrived. Now, "they felt abandoned since no one was there to have them exercise and lead them in activities."

I am concerned about our future commitments toward training physical activity program leaders. In the past, we have turned to institutions of higher learning, and in particular, departments in physical education, to train exercise and physical activity leaders. At a time when the impact of an aging population has suddenly raised questions of preparedness, higher education is undergoing retrenchment. The "golden years" of higher education (the 1960's and early 1970's) was a period in which students were abundant, liberal arts training was in vogue, and capital improvements were massive. During the coming years, higher education may face reductions in student enrollments, layoffs in staff and faculty, and curtailments of programs. For higher education to survive during the 1980's, it must act rather than only react to social and economic distress. An obvious programmatic direction is the training of gerontologists and others concerned with the welfare of an aging society.

Nursing homes, YMCAs and YWCAs, hotels, and senior centers are increasingly seeking professional assistance to initiate programs of physical activity. They frequently turn to the volunteer community help for leadership because universities and colleges have not been responsive to training physical activity leaders to direct older adult programs.

There is some evidence that this picture may be changing. AAHPERD has published a *Physical Fitness Directory,* which is a national directory of colleges and universities that have recently developed programs in physical activity and fitness for the older adult. I have received from a number of institutions outlines of physical education programs with specializations in gerontology that are being initiated. This is encouraging, because a high-risk population engaged in physical activity must be supervised by properly trained personnel.

Required Competencies

The competencies required of future physical activity program leaders working with older adults will vary based on the nature of the program. For example, individuals working in nursing homes may require specialized skills for dealing with our handicapped elderly or the "old-old" (Hooks & Hooks, 1981). Program leaders conducting exercise programs must be certified by the ACSM, which has established training standards for three levels of proficiency: the Exercise Technologist, the Exercise Specialist, and the Program Director. Hiring agencies should ensure that applicants have met ACSM certification requirements. Athletic trainers and activity counselors are also needed on the program "team." Ideally, physical activity programs would adopt a truly integrative approach, seeking a team of professionals to coordinate the physical activity program effort.

Thus, I envision multitrack educational program options in the training of future physical activity leaders. Baccalaureate-level program preparation would seem to be the minimum educational requirement.

Programs at this level would contain courses in the liberal arts core, the professional physical education core, and the gerontology core, and specialization options in exercise physiology/biomechanics, athletic training, counseling, or other relevant fields. Communication skills must also be developed. An important culmination to most programs would be a field-directed training internship at a senior center, YMCA/YWCA, nursing home, or other appropriate site. Clearly, most educational programs must have an interdisciplinary focus. Articles by Leslie (1975) and by Piscopo and Lewis (1977) outline potential baccalaureate-degree program models.

Program specialists should not overlook the potential role of peer-directed leadership. Elderly individuals who are enthusiastic, creative, and concerned should be trained to assist in the direction of physical activity programs. In fact, there may be some interest by these individuals in returning to school to meet certification standards.

Career Opportunities

The myriad of opportunities for the physical activity specialist interested in working with older adults is only limited by one's imagination. Nursing homes, senior centers, and YMCAs and YWCAs have been traditional career sites. I also envision corporations, hotels, health clubs, community recreation departments, private condominiums, and universities seeking professionally trained physical activity specialists. Initially, potential leaders will have to be imaginative and determined in creating new job opportunities. Their actions will markedly influence the receptivity of our society to the need for physical activity specialists among older populations.

The Need for Research Leadership

It is essential to reiterate the need for a concomitant research base to evolve as programs of physical activity for the older adult proliferate. Programs, to be credible, must be guided and documented by scientific evidence. Thus, there is also a need to train future research leaders who have a combined interest in physical activity and gerontology. Higher-education institutions can respond to this need by offering appropriate doctoral degree specializations, by encouraging faculty to "retool" and to seek extramural funding in these areas, by fostering conferences, by creating research institutes dedicated to understanding aging, exercise, and psychomotor skill, and by opening their doors to the older adult. Furthermore, organizations such as the NASPSPA and the ACSM must promote gerontological research.

We must insist upon a universal commitment toward gaining knowledge so that the myths and prejudices about aging are no longer a part of our lives. To do otherwise would be a grave injustice to future generations of older adults.

SUMMARY

In this chapter, I have attempted to synthesize information from previous chapters on what is known about older adult physical activity participation so as to formulate a set of program recommendations. I began the chapter by reviewing a number of prominent physical activity programs around the country that are now available to older adults. These programs are meritorious in recognizing the need for life cycle physical activity participation, but a concomitant research base must evolve to document the practices and outcomes of these programs.

The program principles and recommendations I have developed in this chapter are designed to guide future programs of physical activity for the older adult. These principles and recommendations are not all-inclusive; rather, I sought to highlight those areas, particularly from a psychological perspective, that are most germane to programming. An overriding concern throughout was that we must never forget that older adults are adults first and old second.

I concluded the chapter by urging higher-education institutions to expand their efforts to train individuals interested in directing physical activity programs for the older adult. I outlined briefly the competencies these leaders must have and the career opportunities that await their services. In concluding, I noted that research leaders must also be trained in gerontology and physical activity so that programs of physical activity for the older adult are better documented as we approach the twenty-first century.

REFERENCES

Alliance programs for older Americans. *Journal of Physical Education and Recreation*, 1979, *50*, 31.

American College of Sports Medicine. *Guidelines for graded exercise testing and exercise prescription.* Philadelphia: Lea & Febiger, 1975.

American College of Sports Medicine. The recommended quantity and quality of exercise for developing and maintaining fitness in healthy adults. *Medicine and Science in Sports*, 1978, *10*, vii-x.

Auxter, D. *Perceptual motor development programs for an individually prescribed instructional system.* Unpublished manuscript, Slippery Rock State College, 1971.

Borkan, G.A., & Norris, A.H. Assessment of biological age using a profile of physical parameters. *Journal of Gerontology*, 1980, *35*, 177-184.

Bundschuh, E.L., & Wiegand, R.L. Individualizing motor development within an intact classroom. *WVAHPER Research and Review*, 1975, *1*, 7-8.

Butler, R.N. *Why survive? Being old in America.* New York: Harper & Row, 1975.

Butler, R.N., & Lewis, M.I. *Aging and mental health* (2nd ed.). St. Louis: C.V. Mosby, 1977.

Corbin, D. An exercise program for the elderly. *Physical Educator*, 1981, *38*, 46-49.

deVries, H.A. Fitness after fifty. *Journal of Physical Education and Recreation*, 1976, *47*, 47-49.

Feltz, D.L., & Weiss, M.R. Developing self-efficacy through sport. *Journal of Physical Education, Recreation, and Dance*, 1982, *53*, 24-26.

Fleishman, E.A. *The structure and measurement of physical fitness.* Englewood Cliffs, N.J.: Prentice-Hall, 1964.

Fleishman, E.A. Human abilities and the acquisition of skill. In E.A. Bilodeau (Ed.), *Acquisition of skill.* New York: Academic Press, 1966.

Fleishman, E.A. Performance assessment on an empirically derived task taxonomy. *Human Factors*, 1967, *9*, 349-366.

Fleishman, E.A. On the relation between abilities, learning, and human performances. *American Psychologist*, 1972, *27*, 1017-1032.

Frankel, L.J. Across the nation—Habilitation. In R. Harris & L.J. Frankel (Eds.), *Guide to fitness after 50.* New York: Plenum Press, 1977.

Frankel, L.J., & Richard, B.B. *Be alive as long as you live.* Charleston, W.Va.: Preventicare Publications, 1977.

Franklin, B.A. Motivating and educating adults to exercise. *Journal of Physical Education and Recreation*, 1978, *49*, 13-17.

Garnet, E.D. *Movement is life: A holistic approach to exercise for older adults.* Princeton, N.J.: Princeton Book Co., 1982.

Hattlestad, N.W. Improving the physical fitness of senior adults: A statewide approach. *Journal of Physical Education and Recreation*, 1979, *50*, 29-31.

Hooks, B., & Hooks, E., Jr. Needed: Physical educators on the nursing home team. *Physical Educator*, 1981, *38*, 32-34.

Jable, J.T., & Cheesman, M.J. An exercise project by young adults for senior citizens. *Journal of Physical Education and Recreation*, 1978, *49*, 26-27.

Physical Activity Programs

Kamm, A. Senior olympics. *Journal of Physical Education and Recreation*, 1979, *50*, 32-33.

Leslie, D.K. Fitness programs for the aging. *NAPECW-NCPEAM Briefings*, 1975, 1-10.

Leslie, D.K., & McClure, J.W. *Exercises for the elderly*. Des Moines: Iowa Commission on Aging, 1975.

Leviton, D. Toward a humanistic dimension of HPER. *Journal of Physical Education and Recreation*, 1974, *45*, 41-43.

Leviton, D. The health educator as legislative witness. *Health Education*, 1977, *8*, 33-35.

Lundegren, H.M. Motivation for participation in adult fitness programs. In G.A. Stull (Ed.), *Encyclopedia of physical education, fitness, and sports: Training, environment, nutrition, and fitness*. Salt Lake City: Brighton, 1980.

Martens, R. (Ed.). *Joy and sadness in children's sports*. Champaign, Ill.: Human Kinetics, 1978.

Montoye, H.J. *Physical activity and health: An epidemiologic study of an entire community*. Englewood Cliffs, N.J.: Prentice-Hall, 1975.

Morse, C.E., & Smith, E.L. Physical activity programming for the aged. In E.L. Smith & R.C. Serfass (Eds.), *Exercise and aging: The scientific basis*. Hillside, N.J.: Enslow, 1981.

Ostrow, A.C. Goal-setting behavior and need achievement in relation to a competitive motor activity. *Research Quarterly*, 1976, *47*, 174-183.

Parks, C.J. *The effects of a physical fitness program on body composition, flexibility, heart rate, blood pressure, and anxiety levels of senior citizens*. Unpublished doctoral dissertation, University of Alabama, 1979.

Piscopo, J. Indications and contraindications of exercise and activity for old persons. *Journal of Physical Education and Recreation*, 1979, *50*, 31-34.

Piscopo, J., & Lewis, C.A. Preparing geriatric fitness and recreation specialists. *Journal of Physical Education and Recreation*, 1977, *48*, 48-51.

Rarick, G.L., & Dobbins, D.A. Basic components in the motor performance of children six to nine years of age. *Medicine and Science in Sports*, 1975, *7*, 105-110.

Rarick, G.L., Dobbins, D.A., & Broadhead, G.D. *The motor domain and its correlates in educationally handicapped children*. Englewood Cliffs, N.J.: Prentice-Hall, 1976.

Rarick, G.L., & McQuillan, J.P. *The factor structure of motor abilities of trainable mentally retarded children: Implications for curriculum development* (HEW Report #H 23-3544). Washington, D.C.: U.S. Department of Health, Education and Welfare, 1977.

Shephard, R.J., & Sidney, K.H. Exercise and aging. In R. Hutton (Ed.), *Exercise and sport science reviews* (Vol. 7). Philadelphia: Franklin Institute Press, 1979.

Shivers, J.S., & Fait, H.F. *Recreational service for the aging*. Philadelphia: Lea & Febiger, 1980.

Singer, R.N. *Motor learning and human performance*. New York: Macmillan, 1975.

U.S. Department of Health, Education and Welfare. *The fitness challenge...in the later years* (DHEW Publication No. OHD 75-20802). Washington, D.C.: U.S. Government Printing Office, 1975.

Whitehouse, F.A. Motivation for fitness. In R. Harris & L.J. Frankel (Eds.), *Guide to fitness after 50.* New York: Plenum Press, 1977.

Wiegand, R.L. *A long term analysis of an individualized physical activity program for the mentally retarded.* Paper presented at the American Alliance for Health, Physical Education and Recreation annual convention, Seattle, 1977.

APPENDIX
Bibliography of Training Resources: Physical Exercises for the Elderly

AHDP Fieldhouse. "Smiles: The Adults' Health and Developmental Program." A 29-minute, 16-mm color and sound film on the development of and effects of a program of physical activity, mutual counseling, and learning. Available from: AHDP, Preinkert Fieldhouse, University of Maryland, College Park, MD 20740. Purchase $350, no rental; Audition fee $25 (deductible from purchase price).

Bardone, M. *Yoga and the Older Person.* Seattle: University of Washington, 1975; 12pp. Available from: School of Social Work, University of Washington, Seattle, WA.

Blanda, G. and M. Herskowitz. *Over Forty. Feeling Great and Looking Good.* New York: 1978; 155pp. Available from: Simon and Schuster, Rockefeller Center, 1230 Avenue of the Americas, New York, NY 10020. Purchase price $8.95. Hardback. Presents an easy-to-accomplish fitness program by the former star of the Oakland Raiders football team, George Blanda. Includes exercises and dietary advice.

Canadian Red Cross Society. *Fun and Fitness.* Toronto: September 1974. Available from: Canadian Red Cross Society, 95 Wellesley Street East, Toronto, Ontario M4Y 1H6, Canada. (Revised edition.) Purchase price $1.00.

Christensen, A., S. Rama, and D. Rankin. *Easy Does It Yoga for People Over 60. A Simple Effective Course in Yoga Exercise.* Cleveland Heights, OH: Saraswati Studio, 1976; 56pp. Available from: Saraswati Studio, 12429 Cedar Road, Cleveland Heights, OH 44106.

Dempsey, H. *Recreation Activities for the Older Person: A Beginning Compendium.* Denton, TX: Texas Women's University; 3pp. Available from: College of Health, Physical Education, and Recreation, Texas Women's University, Denton, TX 76201. Lists activities and exercises; has been used in nutrition Project Director's training. Includes one page of wheelchair exercises.

Frankel, L.J. and B.B. Richard. *Be Alive As Long As You Live.* Charleston, WV: Lawrence Frankel Publications, 1977; 256pp. Available from: Preventicare Publications, c/o Lawrence Frankel, Virginia at Brooks Street, Charleston, WV 25301.

Appendix

Hopp, R. *Enjoying the Active Life After Fifty.* Brattleboro, VT: Stephen Greene Press, Inc., 1979; 184pp. Published by Stonewall Press, Inc., 5 Bryon Street, Boston, MA 02108. Discusses the importance of physical activity for middle-aged and older people who wish to maintain or improve their health, with each chapter focusing on a different activity, beginning with the least strenuous and proceeding to more vigorous exercises. References are included.

Kamenetz, Herman L. "Exercises for Older People," *NRTA Journal,* November/December 1977, pp. 44-45.

Kasch, Fred W. and John L. Boyer. *Adult Fitness: Principles and Practices.* Palo Alto, CA: National Press Books, 1968; 147pp. Purchase price about $4.00 in paperback.

King, Frances and William E. Herzing. *Golden Age Exercises.* New York: Crown Publishers, 1968; 134pp. Purchase price about $5.00 to $6.00 in hardback.

Leslie, D.K. and J.W. McClure. *Exercises for the Elderly.* Des Moines: University of Iowa, 1975. Available from: Iowa Commission on the Aging, The Jewett Building, 415 Tenth Street, Des Moines, IA 50319. This booklet contains an annotated collection of exercises for senior citizens and suggestions for organizing and conducting an exercise program. It includes exercise diagrams, self-evaluation questionnaire, exercise record chart, and an annotated bibliography.

Liberty, J. *Adventures with a Modified Physical Fitness Program.* Ann Arbor, MI: University of Michigan, 1975; 9pp. Available from: Institute of Gerontology, University of Michigan, 520 East Liberty Street, Ann Arbor, MI 48109. These nine looseleaf pages describe modified exercises and include diagrams and references.

Maney, J. *A Class in Creative Movement for Residents of an In-Hospital Halfway House Within a Geriatric Therapeutic Community.* Ann Arbor, MI: University of Michigan, 1975; 12pp. Available from: Institute of Gerontology, University of Michigan, 520 East Liberty Street, Ann Arbor, MI 48109. Reports observations about a course in creative movement and includes sample lesson plan.

National Association for Human Development. Active People Over Sixty. (Film.) Available from: National Association for Human Dvelopment, 1750 Pennsylvania Avenue, NW, Washington, DC 20036.

National Association for Human Development. *Basic Exercises for People Over Sixty.* Washington, DC: 1976; 11pp. Available from National Association for Human Development, 1750 Pennsylvania Avenue, NW, Washington, DC 20036.

Appendix

National Association for Human Development. Grow Older, Feel Younger. (Film.) Available from: National Association for Human Development, 1750 Pennsylvania Avenue, NW, Washington, DC 20036.

National Association for Human Development. *Moderate Exercises for People Over Sixty.* Washington, DC: 1976; 12pp. Available from National Association for Human Development, 1750 Pennsylvania Avenue, NW, Washington, DC 20036.

New England Gerontology Center. *Recreation: The Impetus for Social Interaction.* Durham, NH: New England Gerontology Center, 19—. Available from: New England Gerontology Center, 15 Garrison Avenue, Durham, NH 03824.

North Carolina Agricultural Extension Service. *Don't Just Sit There, Exercise.* Raleigh, NC: North Carolina State University, 1972; 5pp.

Paleos, S. *Manual for Recreation/Socialization Techniques for Use With Older Adults.* West Mifflin, PA: Community College of Allegheny County, 1978; 15pp. Available from: Human Services Program, Community College of Allegheny County, South Campus, Community Services, 1750 Clairton Road, Route 885, West Mifflin, PA 15122. A manual developed for participants of one-day workshops, as a reminder of techniques demonstrated; contains activities and exercises involving movement, actor-training techniques, story telling, and music and includes step-by-step descriptions of alignment, yoga, and tai chi exercises.

Peery, Johnette. *Exercises for Retirees.* Milwaukie, OR: 1976. Available from: Johnette Peery, P.O. Box 22081, Milwaukie, OR 97222. Purchase price $1.50, less in quantity. Emphasis on wheelchair exercises.

President's Council on Physical Fitness and Sports. *Adult Physical Fitness.* Washington, DC: Department of Health, Education and Welfare, 1965. Available from: Department of Health and Human Services, President's Council on Physical Fitness and Sports, 330 Independence Avenue, SW, Washington, DC 20201. Purchase price $.75.

President's Council on Physical Fitness and Sports. *The Fitness Challenge in the Later Years. An Exercise Program for Older Americans.* Washington, DC: Department of Health, Education and Welfare, 1975; 28pp. Available from: Department of Health and Human Services, President's Council on Physical Fitness and Sports, 330 Independence Avenue, SW, Washington, DC 20201.

President's Council on Physical Fitness and Sports. *Physical Fitness Research Digest: Exercise and Aging.* H. Harrison Clarke, Ed. Washington, DC: Department of Health, Education and Welfare; 27pp. Available from: Department of

165

Appendix

Health and Human Services, President's Council on Physical Fitness and Sports, 330 Independence Avenue, SW, Washington, DC 20201. May be small charge. Best current abstract of research in field of exercise and aging. Excellent bibliography.

Senior Adult Services, Community Services Division. *Fitness After Fifty*. Livonia, MI: Schoolcraft College, 1977; 7pp. Available from: Schoolcraft College, 18600 Haggerty Road, Livonia, MI 48151.

State of Connecticut. *Sixty-Plus and Physically Fit: Suggested Exercises for Older People*. Hartford, CT: Department of Aging, 1977; 8pp. Available from: Department on Aging, Physical Fitness Committee, 90 Washington Street, Hartford, CT 06115.

Vitale, Frank. *Individualized Fitness Programs*. Englewood Cliffs, NJ: Prentice-Hall, 1973; 292pp. Purchase price $6.00 in paperback.

Wear, R.E. *Fitness, Vitality, and You. Serving the Elderly—The Technique, Part 2*. Durham, NH: New England Gerontology Center; 81pp. Available from: New England Gerontology Center, 15 Garrison Avenue, Durham, NH 03824. Purchase price $5.00 for spiralbound. Funded by Title IV-A of the Older Americans Act. Contains health-oriented exercise program for older adults. Includes text, exercise activities as related to body joints, photographs of exercise progressions, and self-administered pre-exercise questionnaire.

Reprinted with permission of KWIC Training Resources in Aging, Duke University Center for the Study of Aging and Human Development.

Subject Index

Subject Index

Subject Index

Subject Index

Author Index

171

Author Index

Author Index

Author Index

Author Index